Wish you all the luck.

Kumar &
Mitesh.

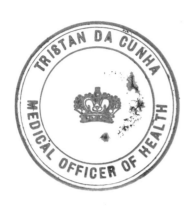

Illustrated Handbook in Local Anaesthesia

SECOND EDITION

Edited by
EJNAR ERIKSSON

Assistant Editor
ANTON DÖBERL

English Translation
VICTOR GOLDMAN
GRAHAM McCARTHY
J. N. MITCHELL

Drawings
POUL BUCKHÖJ

Photographs
MEDICINSK FILMSTUDIO
Upplands Väsby, Sweden

LLOYD-LUKE (Medical Books) LTD.
49 NEWMAN STREET · LONDON

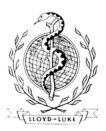

1979

FIRST EDITION .   .   .   1969
SECOND EDITION .   .   .   1979

Printed in Denmark by
I. CHR. SØRENSEN & CO. A/S
Copenhagen

ISBN 085324 145 7

Foreword
to the first edition

The place of local anaesthesia in surgery varies considerably within different hospitals and different countries. Infiltration and spinal anaesthesia are still used relatively often but plexus, epidural anaesthesia and also other peripheral conduction techniques are employed to a varying extent. In recent years regional anaesthesia in many large medical centres has been pushed aside in favour of general anaesthesia. From a medical point of view this is not always desirable even if new narcotic agents and better technical apparatus have become available. In many cases local anaesthesia means the least strain on the patient. Moreover the new local anaesthetic agents which have appeared in the last few years can further motivate a re-evaluation of the role of anaesthesia.

The use of local anaesthetics in areas other than surgery has recently received increased interest. For example continous epidural ananaesthesia has come into much greater use as a possible way of achieving painless childbirth. Preoperative and therapeutic relief of pain is another area where local anaesthetics have received increasing attention. The group of severely ill people who do not receive satisfactory therapy against pain is at present large. The value of local anaesthetics as aids to diagnosis and therapy in various pain conditions will most certainly increase. Certain local anaesthetics have recently been increasingly used in areas other than anaesthesia. Accordingly Xylocaine has been shown to be of value in the treatment of certain forms of cardiac arrythmias and also in epilepsy.

This book is the first collective Swedish work on local anaesthesia.

The idea of publishing a book of this type has been discussed often amongst those Swedish research workers who took an active part in the development and clinical evaluation of the Swedish preparations Xylocaine®, Citanest®, Carbocaine® and Marcaine®. Now that Ejnar Eriksson has taken the initiative, this book will be welcomed especially by anaesthetists and surgeons. By means of the excellent anatomical diagrams, the detailed photography, and its concise text, it will be of great help in training and teaching. This is of considerable value particularly as many anaesthetists have not had the opportunity of making themselves well acquainted with the techniques and possibilities of different forms of regional anaesthesia. May this book therefore stimulate and increase interest in local anaesthesia and regional blockade which on many occasions is a less severe interference with the organism than a long acting narcosis. The book should be of interest for both students and doctors who utilize local anaesthetic agents for operative intervention, therapy and diagnosis both in Sweden and abroad.

TORSTEN GORDH
Professor of Anaesthesia, Karolinska Institute, Stockholm.
Head of the Depts. of Anaesthesia Karolinska Hospital, Stockholm.

Foreword

to the second edition

In 1969 the first edition of the Illustrated Handbook in Local Anaesthesia was published. The idea of a small book with good drawings, illustrative pictures and a short text for practical clinical work in regional analgesia seems to have been a success. All over the world "the little green book" has been used, presumably to the largest extent by newcomers to this very interesting field of anaesthesia. Recently it has been very hard to find a copy of the book, irrespective of the language in which it has been published.

The need for a simple, well-explained handbook in local anaesthesia still exists. It is therefore with great satisfaction I am writing this foreword as it means that anaesthetists now have a new, revised edition of the Illustrated Handbook in Local Anaesthesia. As an introduction to practical clinical regional anaesthesia it will still be very useful and will serve as a complement to the very good and much more complete books, published during the 70-ties.

Department of Anaesthesiology
Linköping University

J. Bertil Löfström
Professor

List of Contributors

VIKTOR VON BAHR
M. D., Former Head of the Dept. of Surgery, Södertälje Hospital, Södertälje, Sweden.

EINAR BOHM
M.D., Professor of Neurosurgery, Uppsala University,
Uppsala. Head of the Dept. of Neurosurgery, Uni-
versity Hospital, Uppsala, Sweden.

SÖREN ENGLESSON
M.D., Head of the Dept. of Anaesthesia, University
Hospital, Uppsala, Sweden.

EJNAR ERIKSSON
M.D., Assistant Professor of Surgery, Karolinska
Institute, Stockholm. Head of the Karolinska Hospi-
tal, Stockholm, Sweden. Editor in Chief.

TOMAS GEJROT
M. D., Assistant Professor of Otorhinolaryngology,
Karolinska Institute, Stockholm. Head of the Dept.
of Otorhinolaryngology, Kristianstad Hospital, Kristianstad, Sweden.

TORSTEN GORDH
M. D., Professor of Anaesthesia, Karolinska Institute,
Stockholm. Former Head of the Depts. of Anaesthe-
sia, Karolinska Hospital, Stockholm, Sweden.

BERTIL LÖFSTRÖM
M.D., Professor of Anaesthesia, Linköping University,
Sweden. Head of the Dept. of Anaesthesia, Regional
Hospital, Linköping, Sweden.

TURE PETRÉN †
M.D., Former Professor of Anatomy, Karolinska Institute, Stockholm, Sweden.

ANNE-MARIE THORN-ALQUIST
M.D., Head of the Dept. of Anaesthesia, University
Hospital, Umeå, Sweden.

BJÖRN WULFING
M.D., Assistant Professor of Ophthalmology, Karolinska Institute, Stockholm, Sweden.

ÅKE WÅHLIN
M.D., L.D.S., Assistant Professor of Anaesthesia,
Karolinska Institute, Stockholm. Head of the Central
Dept. of Anaesthesia, Huddinge Hospital, Stockholm,
Sweden.

ARNE ÅSTRÖM
M.D., Assistant Professor of Physiology, Karolinska
Institute, Stockholm, Sweden. Former Head of the
Dept. of Clinical Research, AB Astra.

Contents

Preface

Ejnar Eriksson

"Teamwork" is now accepted as normal practice in modern medicine. Fundamental research is nowadays carried on by a group of specialists, as a project may easily impinge on several disciplines. There is little place for the lone worker in this field. Similarly the authorship of a medical textbook may well be the concern of a team. Thus this book is the result of co-operation between authors, photographers, artist and editor. Since the illustrations have been produced by an unconventional method, it may be of interest to give a brief account of this procedure.

The subject matter of the illustrations was first decided upon by the editor and each author in turn. A series of trial exposures were then made on Polaroid film and developed immediately. Thus the position of the needle, the composition of the picture, and the lighting could be discussed in detail by the editor, the author, the photographer, and the medical artist before the final photographs were taken. The artist then made sketches while the block was being performed and from the trial exposures on Polaroid film. Thus the drawings and photographs have been built up into an entity. Author and editor, but above all, Professor Ture Petrén of the Department of Anatomy, Karolinska Institute, have checked each drawing. The artist Poul Buckhöj has received tuition in anatomy; moreover, Professor Petrén and Mr. Buckhöj have made special dissections with reference to certain drawings.

Many authors have co-operated in the production of this book. Thus the length and the degree of detail of the different contributions vary. This book does not set out to be a textbook, as the term is usually understood. The object has been, rather, to give an easily accessible general review of the field of usefulness of local anaesthesia, while laying great stress on visually illustrating each procedure. We hope that as such, this book will prove a useful supplement to the excellent textbooks on this subject which are already available.

In this second edition of the book we have added chapters on local anaesthesia in different types of endoscopy since this has proven to be an important indication for the use of local anaesthesia.

The Pharmacology of Local Anaesthetics - Some Observations

ARNE ÅSTRÖM

All the chemical agents which have come into use for the blocking of nerve impulses have the same mode of action. In low concentrations they delay and when present in higher concentrations completely prevent, the migration of ions across the nerve membrane – the normal accompaniment of the transmission of the action potential. This "stabilizing" effect on the cell membrane can be observed not only in nerve cells, but also in the other cells in the body which are capable of excitation. Thus agents of this type have been introduced for the treatment of certain kinds of cardiac arrhythmias, e.g. procaine amide and lignocaine. The blood-brain barrier is freely permeable to local anaesthetics. The rapid depolarizing and repolarizing processes in an epileptic focus are very sensitive to the action of local anaesthetics, therefore lignocaine can be used to treat status epilepticus. On the other hand, toxic doses affect the central nervous system, resulting in convulsions. This may well be explained by the fact that under normal conditions, the inhibitory neurons in the cortex are those most sensitive to the action of local anaesthetics, and are therefore blocked by relatively low concentrations. Consequently, blocking these inhibitory neurons would account for cortical excitation. Higher concentrations will inhibit the central neurons more generally, thus resulting in depression of the respiratory centre, along with other vital centres.

The Local Anaesthetic Action

The blocking action of local anaesthetics on the transmission of nerve impulses may be studied easily using electrophysiological techniques on an isolated nerve, for example, the sciatic nerve of the frog. The determination of latency and recovery gives valuable information concerning the range of usefulness of any particular agent. Usually the effect on an isolated nerve can be well correlated to the physico-chemical properties of that substance.

In vivo the effect of the local anaesthetic is largely dependent on the rate of block perfusion of the tissue injected. Thus absorption is slow from the spinal canal, while in the region of the jaw, for example, it is so rapid that a vasoconstrictor must be added to most local anaesthetics if an adequate frequency and duration of effect is to be obtained. Moreover, different local anaesthetics are absorbed at differing rates from the same tissues, because they influence the local circulation to a varying degree. The addition of a vasoconstrictor in order to delay absorption and thus reduce the risk of toxic side effects is particularly important if the local anaesthetic agent is rapidly absorbed (e.g. amethocaine).

The different nerve fibres are blocked in a fixed order. Fine fibres are easier to block than the coarser ones. Thus sensitivity is lost first (pain and temperature before touch) and motor function last. A local anaesthetic with considerable power of penetration is required to block major nerve trunks.

The effect of the local anaesthetic is determined by the concentration attained within the nerve. The main characteristics of the concentration curve may be seen in fig. 2.

Immediately after injection, the local anaesthetic is present in excess in the envi-

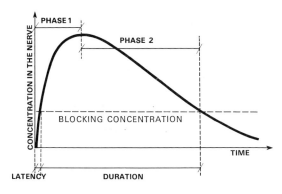

Fig. 2

ronment of the nerve and therefore rapidly penetrates into the nerve trunk. (Phase I). Penetration may be facilitated either by increasing the concentration of the solution injected, or, in highly vascularized tissue, by maintaining a high concentration around the nerve by means of a vasoconstrictor. Both the latent period and the maximum concentration attained in the nerve are determined by the course of Phase I. The speed at which the concentration in the nerve falls below the level required for nerve block (Phase II) is determined partly by the drug's affinity for the lipoprotein constituent of the nerve and partly by the concentration gradient across the cell membrane. The addition of a vasoconstrictor would seem to increase primarily the maximum concentration reached during Phase I. However, it also delays the removal of the drug by the circulation from the environment of the nerves during Phase II.

It is difficult from experiments performed on laboratory animals to assess the significance of the various factors which determine the behaviour of a local anaesthetic agent with different types of nerve block. So every new local anaesthetic must be evaluated clinically, with regard to its range of application, choice of a suitable concentration, and the optimum strength of a vasoconstrictor, should such be required.

Toxicity

As in the case of all drugs, the toxicity of local anaesthetics must be assessed with regard to their effect. Clinical tolerance depends to a large extent on the rate of uptake by the circulation from the site of administration. Should this be slow, the rate of detoxification is of particular significance.

The toxic effects of a local anaesthetic primarily involve the cardiovascular and central nervous systems. With rapid intravenous administration, central nervous system toxicity is well correlated to the specific local anaesthetic activity of the agent concerned. This may be determined by using an isolated nerve preparation. Thus with intravenous administration, the more potent compound lignocaine gives rise to central nervous system symptoms more readily than prilocaine or mepivacaine. With tissue infiltration or nerve block, on the other hand, the local anaesthetic action varies because different agents are absorbed at different rates from the site of administration. There is then but little correlation between the local anaesthetic action, as measured in this way and acute intravenous toxicity. The addition of a vasoconstrictor reduces the uptake of lignocaine by the circulation more than that of prilocaine or mepivacaine. When the blood concentration is rising relatively slowly, due to absorption from a tissue depot, or with slow intravenous administration, the rate of detoxification and differences in distribution to the different body-tissues significantly affect tolerance and toxicity.

Cardiovascular side-effects are sometimes very alarming. With the dosage recommended, local anaesthetics reduce myocardial excitability which makes lignocaine, for example, most suitable for the treatment of ventricular arrhythmias. The same pharmacological mode of action, nevertheless, causes a certain prolongation of conduction-time, which occasionally can lead to varying degrees of block with a fall in blood-pressure. With very high blood concentrations, depression of the myocardium and dilatation of the peripheral resistance-vessels can occur.

Useful information about the toxicity of local anaesthetics and the pattern of their detoxification may be obtained from animal experiments. But clinical tolerance must be assessed on human subjects, by pharmacological tests and large-scale clinical trials. Not the least reason for this is the considerable species-differences in the way animals break down and inactivate drugs. Species differences also apply to local toxicity, i.e. local irritation.

Different Local Anaesthetic Agents

Local anaesthetics are, as a general rule, either esters or amides with the following general formulae:

$$H_2N \langle \rangle COO \ R \ N \langle {R_1 \atop R_2}$$ $$\langle \rangle NH \ CO \ R \ N \langle {R_1 \atop R_2}$$

Ester Type	Amide Type

R, R_1, R_2 = Alkyl group containing 1-3 C-atoms

Esters have the pharmaceutical disadvantage of being less stable in solution. The best-known representatives of this group are procaine and amethocaine.

Procaine has limited powers of tissue-penetration and to a very large extent has been replaced by the newer agents of the amide group.

Amethocaine has retained its position as a satisfactory agent for spinal anaesthesia. Amethocaine is absorbed extraordinarily rapidly from mucous membranes (for example, of the tracheo-bronchial tree) and the risk of

toxic side-effects is therefore great, thus limiting its usefulness. If absorption of this agent is delayed by the addition of a vasoconstrictor, when used in regional blocks, a very long-lasting effect will result.

Local anaesthetics of the amide type are remarkably stable and solutions prepared from these substances may be sterilized repeatedly by autoclaving. Apparently they also cause significantly fewer sensitivity reactions than para-amino benzoic acid derivatives (procaine and amethocaine). Lignocaine, prilocaine, mepivacaine, bupivacaine and etidocaine belong to the amide group.

Lignocaine has a remarkably good power of penetration and so produces adequate blocks in regions where procaine has proved unsatisfactory (brachial plexus, epidural space etc.). Lignocaine has therefore become the most widely used local anaesthetic agent in most parts of the world. Both prilocaine and mepivacaine are comparable clinically with lignocaine in their effects.

Prilocaine is absorbed more slowly than lignocaine, and so is less dependent on the addition of a vasoconstrictor. This slower absorption results in the nerve tissue being more saturated with prilocaine and the *"in vivo"* effect is as good as that of lignocaine, in spite of the fact that its local anaesthetic potency, as measured on an isolated nerve, is somewhat lower than that of lignocaine. The lower effect on the isolated nerve corresponds with a lower acute toxicity on the central nervous system. Even after intravenous injection, prilocaine results in a lower blood level than lignocaine, due to differences in distribution and peripheral uptake. Prilocaine is broken down mainly by amidases in the liver, and with considerably greater rapidity than lignocaine or mepivacaine. If therefore toxic symptoms should appear following overdosage, they are only transient.

Mepivacaine resembles prilocaine in that its activity, as assessed on the isolated nerve, is lower than that of lignocaine; again, this disadvantage *in vivo* is compensated by slower absorption. Its need of added vasoconstrictor is also less than that of lignocaine. Mepivacaine is not metabolized as rapidly as prilocaine, so should toxic symptoms appear, they will be of longer duration.

Bupivacaine is chemically related to mepivacaine. However, the potency and the toxicity is increased. Bupivacaine has a long duration of action. In several clinical applications, bupivacaine produces adequate analgesia with only moderate degree of motor blockade. Vasoconstrictors combined with bupivacaine seem to be of less importance for the duration than when combined with e.g. lignocaine.

Etidocaine is chemically related to lignocaine but has a longer duration of action. Etidocaine has a more rapid onset of action than bupivacaine. In many clinical applications it produces a marked motor blockade. Although etidocaine like bupivacaine has a high potency, it has been found to have an adequate margin of safety. This is, at least in part, probably due to a rapid redistribution of the drug.

For further information consult textbooks e.g. Covino, Vassallo, Local Anaesthetics, Mechanisms of action and clinical use (1976 by Grune & Stratton Inc., N.Y.), de Jong, Local Anaesthetics (1977 by C. C. Tomas, Springfield, Illinois).

Dosage and Maximum Doses

The concentration and volume of solutions of local anaesthetics required to give satisfactory results vary widely. Lignocaine 0.25-0.5 % gives completely satisfactory results with infiltration anaesthesia, while motor block in conjunction with epidural anaesthesia requires a concentration of 1.5-2 %. The risk of side effects also varies with the site and mode of administration. Absorption from the tracheo-bronchial tree is so rapid that it is comparable with slow intravenous injection, while absorption from the urinary bladder is significantly slower, the difference being at least tenfold. It is thus apparent that the stating of generally applicable maximum doses is of limited value. How often a well-tolerated single dose may be repeated in the course of a couple of hours is also very variable for different drugs and often inadequately investigated. The addition of a vasoconstrictor usually increases clinical tolerance in all sites of administration except in the tracheobronchial tree and on intravenous injection. However, this increase in tolerance varies with the site of injection, as well as with the nature and concentration of the agent.

As an example of maximum recommended doses the following Swedish figures* may be given:

Bupivacaine without adrenaline	150 mg
Bupivacaine with adrenaline	150 mg
Etidocaine without adrenaline	300 mg
Etidocaine with adrenaline	400 mg
Lignocaine without adrenaline	200 mg
Lignocaine with adrenaline	500 mg
Mepivacaine without adrenaline	350 mg
Mepivacaine with adrenaline	350 mg
Prilocaine without adrenaline	400 mg
Prilocaine with adrenaline	600 mg

* These apply to an adult patient of 70 kg body weight.

Introduction to Local Anaesthesia

Ejnar Eriksson

If possible, regional anaesthesia should be performed taking the same sterile precautions as those taken during surgical operations.

The site of administration must be prepared and draped. Sterile syringes must be used, preferably those from a ready-packed sterile set containing all the equipment required. A detailed list of contents, preferably illustrated, facilitates the preparation of the various sets by the operating theatre staff (fig. 3). Whenever possible the anaesthetist should wear cap, mask, theatre clothing, and sterile gloves (fig. 4). The only exceptions are certain minor outpatient procedures.

An indwelling intravenous needle or catheter should be inserted into a readily avail-

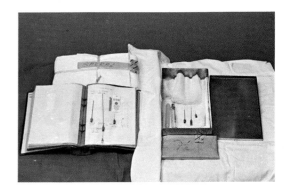

Fig. 3

Resuscitation Equipment:
 – the minimum compatible with safety.
1. Table or trolley on which the patient can be placed in the head-down (Trendelenburg) position immediately.
2. An oxygen cylinder, a self-inflating bag, a one-way valve (e.g. Ruben) and a suitable face-piece for intermittent positive pressure ventilation.
3. Suction apparatus and catheters.
4. Nasal and oro-pharyngeal airways or ideally equipment for intubation.
5. A short-acting barbiturate (i.e. thiopentone) for intravenous administration, succinyl choline in ampoules.
6. A sympathomimetic (e.g. methoxamine, metaraminol). (cf. page 18-19)

able peripheral vein in all cases other than minor outpatient procedures. This will enable immediate treatment of any complication.

When paraesthesia has been elicited the needle must be withdrawn a millimetre or two prior to the injection. Resistance to injection combined with paraesthesia is likely to be due to intraneural injection.

Aspiration is essential before all injections. If the needle is placed in situ prior to attaching the syringe, blood may ooze from the hub indicating that a vessel has been penetrated. However, this must not replace aspiration once the syringe is attached. Accidental rapid intravascular injection of a dose which is usual for many procedures would be sufficient to produce severe toxic reactions. Once the local has been administered the patient must not be left alone. Ideally the anaesthetist should stay with his patient. When this is not possible an experienced nurse should be detailed for this purpose.

It is unwise to persuade a patient to undergo surgery under local anaesthesia if he prefers a general anaesthetic, unless his condition necessitates such a technique. A history of unfavourable reactions during local anaesthesia is a relative contraindication. If possible, another method of anaesthesia should be selected in such cases.

Resuscitation equipment must be immediately available.

Fig. 4

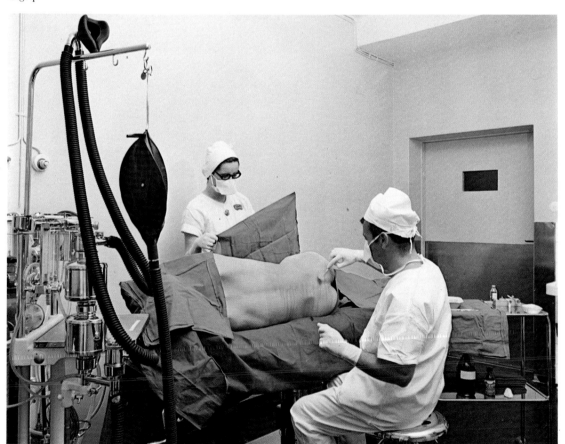

Complications and Their Treatment

Torsten Gordh

All local anaesthetic drugs are, to a greater or lesser extent, toxic substances, and for that reason maximum doses are stated for each agent. Two kinds of toxic reactions can be distinguished – either local or general.

Local Complications

These occur at the site of injection and include oedema, inflammation, abscess-formation, necrosis and gangrene. Infective complications are almost invariably caused by neglect of sterile precautions. Tissue-reactions in the form of oedema have been observed mainly in dental practice and have been shown to be due to metallic ions such as copper, zinc or nickel having gained access to the local anaesthetic solution. Such local reactions have been eliminated by avoiding the use of syringes and containers made of these metals.

A much more serious complication is a tissue reaction due to the vasoconstrictor contained in the local anaesthetic solution. The injection of a depot containing an excessive quantity of adrenaline can lead to necro-

sis and gangrene due to tissue ischaemia. Cases of gangrene have also been described following regional block of a digit or of the penis. Therefore vasoconstrictors and particularly the simultaneous use of a tourniquet to ensure a bloodless field, are contraindicated in tissues containing end-arteries, such as in the fingers, toes and penis. Should a typical ischaemic demarcation zone with inflamed margins appear in the skin, for example, after the injection of local anaesthetic, excision of the affected area should be considered, since necrosis calling for secondary excision and skin-grafting may occur. If local tissue damage due to vasoconstrictors be suspected, one should not fail to use vasodilators and/or sympathetic blocks.

Injuries caused by the needle used for injection should also be considered under this heading. Such injuries may consist of haematoma formation, nerve injury and pneumothorax – as, for example, following a brachial plexus block. Serious complications – both local and general – have followed the inadvertent injection of such toxic solutions as alcohol, formalin, hydrochloric acid and mercuric chloride in mistake for solutions of local anaesthetic.

General Complications

General complications are the outcome of the effect of the local anaesthetic on the various systems of the body. They are usually classified according to their clinical manifestations, e.g. "neurological" or "cardiovascular" reactions. One may also speak of "immediate" or "delayed" reactions, the former being rapidly progressive with primary cardiovascular failure, while the latter follow a slower course leading to respiratory failure. Sometimes symptoms involving the central nervous system predominate – convulsions, loss of consciousness and respiratory depression – sometimes the effect on the cardiovascular system predominates – circulatory failure being the primary symptom.

EFFECT ON THE CENTRAL NERVOUS SYSTEM

It has been demonstrated experimentally (Steinhaus 1957) that the cerebral cortex and higher centres are stimulated by local anaesthetics, while the medulla and pons are depressed. In the former case signs of stimulation manifest themselves, i.e. *tremors or convulsions* – in the latter case *respiratory depression* is the salient factor. Probably the cause of death in these cases is medullary depression, leading to respiratory failure.

EFFECT ON THE CARDIOVASCULAR SYSTEM

The cardiovascular effects of local anaesthetics are characterised by a *fall in blood pressure* and a direct *depression of the myocardium* affecting both conduction and contraction. The interesting work by Steinhaus (1957) on rabbits demonstrates the primary reactions from the central nervous system as well as the cardiovascular system. He injected identical doses of cocaine in the aorta, both above and at the level of the origin of the coronary arteries. In the former case typical convulsions and respiratory arrest resulted both with small changes in blood pressure; in the latter the result was a severe fall in blood pressure with weak heart action, but without respiratory arrest. Naturally there is a summation of effect on the different systems, but often one of them predominates. The effect on the heart is certainly the most serious one.

Fig. 5 is a typical tracing from the author's investigation of the effect of the intravenous injection of lignocaine. The respiration, blood pressure, heart volume, aortic flow and the central venous pressure have been recorded in rabbits while breathing spontaneously under urethane anaesthesia. (Gordh 1964 a, b) The injection of 4 mg/kg into the external

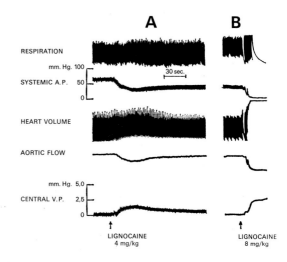

Fig. 5

Respiration, blood pressure, heart volume and central venous pressure in a rabbit under light urethane anaesthesia: A following a rapid i.v. injection of 4 mg./kg. of lignocaine; B following a lethal dose (8 mg./kg.) as a rapid i.v. injection shortly after the first dose. At A the heart volume is somewhat increased, the respiration is virtually unchanged. At B there is maximum cardiac dilatation before subsequent respiratory arrest.

jugular vein resulted in a transitory fall in blood pressure and aortic blood flow, while the heart dilated and central venous pressure rose. When a lethal dose was injected, the result was rapid cardiovascular failure with maximum dilatation of the heart and respiratory arrest. Thus a direct myocardial depression would seem to be the dominant toxic reaction in cases of cardiovascular collapse.

PSYCHOGENIC REACTIONS

These cannot be grouped with toxic reactions to local anaesthetics, but they ought to be mentioned, since the symptoms can sometimes be similar. Pain and fear can give rise, reflexly, to vaso-motor disturbances; pallor, nausea, cold sweating and fall in blood pressure leading to neurogenic syncope. These reactions usually occur when the patient is in the upright position. Thus they are more common in out-patient practice, specially in the dental chair and in otolaryngological practice. Cerebral hypoxia with loss of consciousness and even anoxic tremors and convulsions may occur before the patient can be placed in the horizontal position. Treatment consists in rapid lowering of the patient's head and thorax, and possibly the administration of oxygen.

METHAEMOGLOBINAEMIA

Certain drugs may give rise to methaemoglobin (ferrihaemoglobin) formation. One of these drugs is prilocaine when administered in large doses. Due to the rapid breakdown to pharmacologically less active substances, the clinical toxicity of prilocaine is very low. However, one of the metabolites produces ferrihaemoglobin. This reaction, which after a single dose of 600 mg. involves approximately 4-6 % of the total haemoglobin, is spontaneously reversible.

Following high doses of prilocaine (e.g. in continuous epidural anaesthesia) cyanosis may sometimes be observed as a symptom of methaemoglobinemia. In such cases, signs of methaemoglobin formation can also be observed in the newborn, which may be of differential diagnostic significance versus hypoxic cyanosis. Otherwise the formation of ferrihaemoglobin due to prilocaine is clinically insignificant. In patients with severely impaired oxygen carrying capacity (e.g. severe anaemia) the disadvantage of large doses of prilocaine reducing the amount of haemoglobin available for oxygen transport must be balanced against the higher toxicity and less favourable safety margin of other local anaesthetic agents.

Since prilocaine-induced ferrihaemoglobin formation is spontaneously reversible there is, in principle, no need for treatment. Intravenously administered methylene blue (1 mg. per kg of body weight) prevents the formation of ferrihaemoglobin; already formed ferrihaemoglobin can if considered desirable be treated with this dose of methylene blue with the effect that cyanosis disappears within 15 minutes.

Discussion of the Treatment of Toxic Reactions

The most important measure is to ensure adequate oxygenation by artificial respiration with oxygen. Should marked tremors or convulsions appear, small intravenous doses of a short-acting barbiturate, such as sodium thiopentone, are recommended. Their site of action is located chiefly in the region of the pons, where they produce a functional decerebration (Gordh 1952) by blocking the efferent impulses from the cerebral cortex, thus convulsions cease. *This is the only function of the barbiturates in this context.* At the same time it must be realised that the respiratory depressant action of the barbiturate will be added to the depression already present. Consequently it is even more essential to continue lung inflation with the addition of oxygen. If the patient be unconscious, convulsions can also be abolished by injecting a short-acting muscle relaxant (e.g. succinyl choline) which acts peripherally. Naturally, paralysis of the respiratory muscles must then be taken into account. If an intravenous injection is not possible the muscle relaxant should be given intramuscularly immediately. Myocardial depression if present will be aggravated by hypoxia or anoxia. Therefore it is essential in any event to commence treatment by artificial ventilation with oxygen. Circulatory depression may require the administration of a sympathomimetic drug intravenously as a bolus injection or drip. Should cardiac arrest be suspected, external cardiac massage should be instituted immediately.

1. Treat respiratory depression with oxygen and artificial respiration (intubation).
2. Treat circulatory depression with oxygen and artificial ventilation + a head-down tilt + blood pressure raising drugs intravenously.

   Should cardiac arrest be suspected, commence external cardiac massage immediately.
3. Treat convulsions with oxygen and artificial ventilation + small intravenous doses (50-150 mg.) of a short-acting barbiturate such as sodium thiopentone. Succinyl choline too can be used to stop convulsions, if the patient has lost consciousness.

Conclusions

Potentially fatal toxic reactions are uncommon, provided that the dose injected is related to the patient's age, body weight and general condition.

Most toxic reactions occur following the use of local anaesthetic agents in highly vascularized tissue, where re-absorption into the blood stream takes place more readily than from a subcutaneous depot. This is particularly true for the throat and the air-ways, as well as the perineum and the urethra. However, toxic reactions may also occur following normal infiltration anaesthesia and nerve block (Gordh, 1946). Every doctor who uses local anaesthetic agents in any form should be aware of the risks involved and how reactions should be treated.

If toxic reactions occur, they are usually due to overdosage, accidental intravascular injection or the administration of a normal dose to an over-sensitive patient. True allergy is indeed rare when the amide group of local anaesthetic agents is employed (e.g. lignocaine). Reactions – especially cardiovascular – can appear surprisingly quickly and without real warning, consequently a patient must never be left unsupervised. This is especially true following local anaesthesia in a highly vascular region, e.g. the throat or after a stellate ganglion block. Furthermore regional anaesthesia should be administered in a place where resuscitation measures such as artificial ventilation with oxygen, a head down tilt, intubation and external cardiac massage can be instituted immediately. An intravenous barbiturate and succinyl choline should be available to control convulsions. Should an intravenous anaesthesic agent or succinyl choline be given, the resulting condition is one of respiratory failure and must be treated accordingly.

Further, the least possible volume of the weakest effective solution should be used. A 2 % solution of lignocaine has been used in far too many cases, when a 0.25 %, 0.5 %, 1.0 % or perhaps 1.5 % solution would have done equally well. The 2 % or stronger solutions are very seldom required, and should be used only when specially indicated. The amount of adrenaline, too, must be considered, as well as the risk of mistakes in concentration or even the composition of the solution.

Our local anaesthetic drugs are now so good as regards latency, potency and duration that research has been directed primarily towards agents with a lower toxicity.

Premedication
- a Survey

Bertil Löström

The Functions of Premedication are as follows:

1. To sedate the patient both during the performance of the block and during the ensuing operation. Surgery may be prolonged, in which case the patient will have to remain composed for a long time.
2. To give the patient pain-relief, should such be required due to fracture or some other trauma, in order to make transport, waiting etc. more comfortable.
3. To reduce reflexes mediated via the cholinergic nerves (i.e. reduce formation of secretions and vaso-vagal reflexes respectively).
4. To minimise, if possible, toxic reactions from the local anaesthetic agent.

These last two functions are usually of less significance.

General Remarks

It is important that the patient feels at ease during the administration of the local anaesthetic and during the operation. The most important factor is that the patient has confidence in both anaesthetist and surgeon. Pre-medication is not generally necessary prior to short operations. On the other hand, more complicated regional techniques and surgical procedures of longer duration call for adequate sedation. Drugs to be used are diazepam or barbiturates – e.g. pentobarbitone.

Furthermore, the technique used by the anaesthetist is very important. The use of fine-gauge needles and gentle injection of the local anaesthetic solution is of the greatest importance. In addition, the patient must be told beforehand what he has to expect.

In cases of painful injuries the patient should receive analgesic drugs intramuscularly, or better still, intravenously in small doses prior to being transferred to the operating theatre. However, analgesics are inadequate in compensating for incomplete local anaesthesia. Premedication containing analgesic drugs interferes considerably with the patient's sensation of paraesthesia, which is necessary if a high success rate of certain types of nerve blocks is to be achieved.

The patient often believes that he feels pain, when in fact it is sensation of touch or pressure in the operative field, or the sight and sound of the surgeon at work which is upsetting him. Here again diazepam, given in small doses, intravenously, are of the greatest value.

Belladonna preparations are used to reduce vagal reflexes and salivary secretion respectively during anaesthesia. In the author's experience, some patients, particularly in the younger age groups, readily show signs of vaso-vagal reflexes, such as bradycardia, low blood pressure or nausea; symptoms which are eliminated by adequate preoperative atropinisation. Thus it may be justified to include either atropine or scopolamine in the premedication. However, as a rule belladonna drugs should not be given to patients undergoing surgery under local anaesthesia. If a vaso-vagal syncope occurs or has occurred on a previous occasion during local anaesthesia, atropinisation is indicated; preferably intravenously immediately before the block. In the same way, atropine may be given to patients undergoing spinal or epidural anaesthesia in order to counteract bradycardia, as well as prior to supplemental general anaesthesia. The principal disadvantage of atropine is dryness of the mouth. In addition it has been reported to lower arterial oxygen tension in the higher age groups. Scopolamine on the other hand may cause undesirable excitation if used in large doses. In careful dosage (cf. scheme C) it produces sedation and a certain degree of amnesia.

In major surgery the anaesthetist must be prepared to administer supplemental general anaesthesia, particularly if the surgery involved turns out to be more extensive or of longer duration than was anticipated. For this reason too, it may be an advantage to include atropine or scopolamine in the premedication.

Barbiturate or diazepam are of great value in stopping convulsions caused by local anaesthetics. On the other hand, reasonable doses of barbiturate given as premedication are not likely to reduce the incidence of such convulsions. Heavy premedication will in fact augment the depressant toxic effect which may occur following large doses of local anaesthetic agents. Therefore pentobarbitone or thiopentone should not be injected intravenously until local anaesthesia is well established, thus normally at a time when the peak concentration of the drug in the plasma has been passed (i.e. after 20–30 minutes). As a rule, this will be when surgery is about to commence.

Suggested Scheme for Premedication of Adult Patients

The anaesthetist should examine the patient on the day before operation and at the same time decide on suitable premedication for individual requirements. The following schemes will serve as a guide for an average adult.

A. Diazepam 10 mg. orally on the evening before operation. Diazepam 5-10 mg. orally, possibly combined with atropine (0.5 mg.) or scopolamine (0.40-0.6 mg.) given intramuscularly or subcutaneously approximately one hour before the administration of the local anaesthetic.
If further sedation is required, repeated small intravenous doses of diazepam (2.5-5 mg.) or of thiopentone (25-50 mg.) may be given before and/or during the administration of the block as well as during surgery.

B. The following scheme may be used for the relief of pain, e.g. due to fractures: Pethidine 50 or 100 mg. is diluted with isotonic saline to 10 or 20 ml. solution, respectively. 2 ml. of this dilute solution is given intravenously in repeated doses at intervals of a few minutes, until the required degree of analgesia is obtained. Changes in pulse, blood pressure, respiration and general condition must be carefully observed. As an alternative, 1 ml. of the standard solution of morphine and scopolamine (each ml. containing 10 mg. morphine hydrochloride and 0.4 mg. scopolamine hydrobromide) may be diluted to 10 ml. and administered as above.

C. The standard solution of morphine and scopolamine (each ml. containing 10 mg. morphine hydrochloride and 0.4 mg. scopolamine hydrobromide) may also be given intramuscularly according to the following scheme:

Age (years)	Morphine-scopolamine (standard-solution)
20-40	1.0 ml. (females)
	1.5 ml. (males)
40-55	1.0 ml.
55-70	0.5 ml.
>70	0.25 ml.

D. Pentobarbitone in doses of 50-100 mg. orally given 1½ hours before the administration of local anaesthesia, followed ½ hour later by morphine-scopolamine intramuscularly according to the above scheme produces powerful sedation and decreases to a large extent the patient's memory of being moved to the operating theatre.

Suggested Scheme for Premedication in Children

A. Diazepam in a solution for rectal administration in a dose of 0.2-0.3 mg./kg. of body weight.

B. (Premedication according to R.M. Smith*)

Age (years)	Body weight (kg.)	Pento-barbitone	Morphine	Atropine or sco-polamine
1	10	50 mg.	1.0 mg.	0.2 mg.
2	12	60 mg.	1.5 mg.	0.3 mg.
4	16	90 mg.	3.0 mg.	0.3 mg.
6	21	100 mg.	4.0 mg.	0.4 mg.
8	25	100 mg.	5.0 mg.	0.4 mg.
10	30	100 mg.	5.0 mg.	0.4 mg.

As a rule these drugs are administered intramuscularly.

Special Remarks

In *interventions in the region of the neck* diazepam plus a small dose of pethidine in

* "Anesthesia for Infants and Children", Ed. 3, The C. V. Mosby Comp. 1968.

addition to a belladonna preparation gives a good sedation and a decreased "sensitivity" in the throat.

In *obstetrics,* premedication – whether barbiturates or morphine derivatives be used – will cause foetal depression. The vitality of the newborn child will be decreased in those cases. (Nalorphine may be injected through the umbilical vein as an antidote). In this context it does not seem to make a significant difference whether pethidine has been given either several hours or a relatively short time before delivery.

Geriatric patients usually require little or no premedication. It is of particular importance to avoid large doses of barbiturates which frequently cause restlessness. Similarly significant doses of atropine and particularly scopolamine may cause excitation in older patients. Promethazine 25 mg. or chloral hydrate 1 G. orally the night before in these patients will provide a good night's sleep and may eliminate the need for premedication in its true sense.

Certain cases call for special consideration of the *underlying disease.* Thus patients suffering from myxoedema are extremely sensitive to depressive drugs. In *porphyria* barbiturates may cause a porphyric attack. Patients suffering from *thyrotoxicosis* or *cardiac disease* usually require heavier premedication than a correspondingly healthy individual. If minor surgical interventions – which can easily be done under regional block (e.g. nerve block at the ankle, p. 112) – are to be undertaken in patients with *diabetes mellitus* no premedication should be used nor should the patient be fasting. The patient should receive his normal dose of insulin.

Infiltration Anaesthesia - General Remarks

EJNAR ERIKSSON

The majority of minor surgical operations, such as the excision of small tumours, incision of abscesses, the suturing of wounds, etc. may be performed under infiltration anaesthesia. The subcutaneous branches of the respective sensory nerves are anaesthetized by the injection of a local anaesthetic drug into the cutaneous and subcutaneous tissues.

TECHNIQUE

To induce anaesthesia for the removal of minor defects in the skin, such as cutaneous or subcutaneous tumours, the drug is infiltrated fanwise from two points, one above and one below the tumour (fig. 6).

Many clinicians consider an injection into infected tissue to be contraindicated. How-

Fig. 6

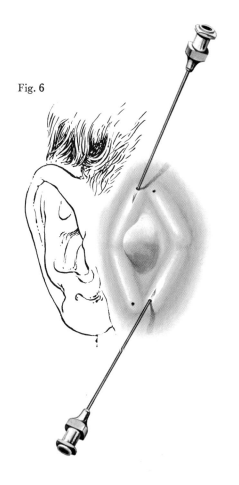

Fig. 7

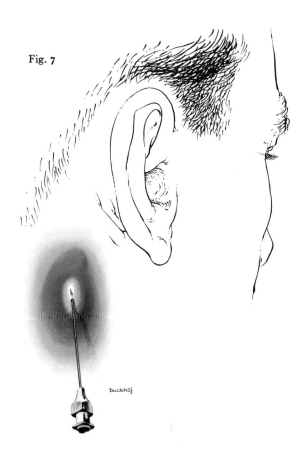

buckhöj

ever, in the author's experience the injection of a minute quantity of local anaesthetic agent with a fine gauge needle, made where the abscess is pointing, is without risk and at times the simplest and most suitable form of anaesthesia. A slow injection (to minimize pain) of 0.3 to 0.5 ml. of 0.5-1.0 % lignocaine or prilocaine produces an intracutaneous weal of sufficient size for painless incision (fig. 7). The usual field block may well give rise to a greater spread of bacteria than a weal over the point of an abscess.

A combination of both local infiltration and light general anaesthesia may be used for more extensive operations, such as fractures of the neck of femur, laparotomy on bad risk cases etc. (cf. Infiltration Anaesthesia for Caesarean Section, page 51). The technique consists of fan-shaped injections of local anaesthetic solution infiltrating the various layers of tissue to be incised.

DOSAGE

The dose depends on the extent of the operation. For infiltration anaesthesia, dilute solutions may be used: lignocaine or prilocaine 0.25-0.5 %, with a vasoconstrictor. When large volumes are used the total amount of vasoconstrictor injected together with the local anaesthetic solution must be taken into account. Necrosis of the wound edges has been observed following the injection of very large volumes (150 ml.) of lignocaine 0.5 % with adrenaline, because of severe tissue ischaemia, due to the adrenaline. Therefore the adrenaline concentration should not exceed 1:200.000, at any rate for major infiltrations (cf. p. 16).

Minor excisions and incisions:
5-30 ml. lignocaine 0.25-0.5 % with adrenaline 1:200.000
5-30 ml. prilocaine 0.25-0.5 % with adrenaline 1:250.000

More extensive excisions – as well as infiltration prior to operative incision:
30-200 ml. lignocaine 0.25 % with adrenaline 1:200.000
30-100 ml. lignocaine 0.5 % adrenaline 1:200.000
30-240 ml. prilocaine 0.25 % with adrenaline 1:250.000
30-120 ml. prilocaine 0.5 % with adrenaline 1:250.000

INDICATIONS

Infiltration anaesthesia is indicated whenever good operative conditions can be obtained with a moderate quantity of local anaesthetic agent because the risk of complications might well be comparatively less than following major nerve blocks or general anaesthesia.

CONTRAINDICATIONS

There are no special contraindications. In tissues supplied by endarteries i.e. toes, fingers and penis, local anaesthetic solution should be used without vasoconstrictor – or at any rate in very low concentrations (adrenaline 1:200.000 at the most).

Infiltration anaesthesia should be avoided in apprehensive patients, especially those who claim to have reacted unfavourably to local anaesthesia previously. Furthermore local anaesthesia should not be used for major procedures in small children.

Local Anaesthesia of the Scalp

Einar Bohm

Most intracranial operations are currently performed under general anaesthesia. However, in acute head injuries it may sometimes be necessary to operate under local anaesthesia. Even when general anaesthesia is routine, local infiltration is often used in the skin flap since this allows a lighter plane of general anaesthesia to be employed. Lignocaine or prilocaine 0.5 % with the addition of adrenaline is most suitable since this results in a reduction of bleeding from the highly vascular soft tissue. The solution is first deposited in the subcutaneous tissue *above* the epicranial aponeurosis, where the nerves and vessels are situated (fig. 8), followed by an infiltration *beneath* the aponeurosis. If the tissue underneath the epicranial aponeurosis alone is infiltrated, neither satisfactory anaesthesia nor the haemostatic effect of adrenaline will be obtained.

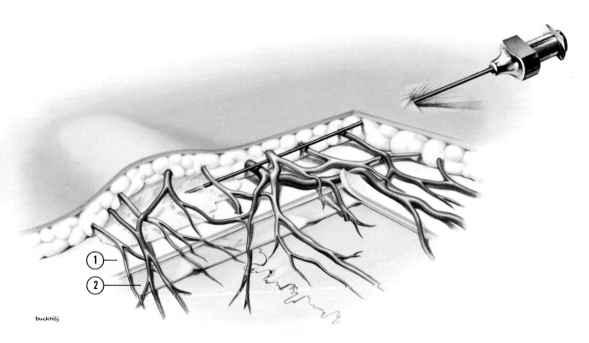

buckhöj

Fig. 8
1. Epicranial aponeurosis
2. Epicranium

Surface Anaesthesia of the Cornea and Conjunctiva

Björn Wulfing

Instillation of local anaesthetic solution (lignocaine 4 %, prilocaine 4 %, tetracaine 1 %, oxibuprocaine 0.2 %) may be performed in two ways (fig. 9, 10).

1-2 drops are sufficient for each instillation; even then excess solution will run from the outer canthus. The *number of instillations* is of far greater significance than the amount administered for each instillation.

TONOMETRY

The cornea is relatively easy to anaesthetize, because of its avascularity. Anaesthesia adequate for *tonometry* usually requires only one instillation. However, it is better to repeat the instillation after an interval of $1/2$-1 minute. Normally the first instillation causes a little smarting and blepharospasm. When the discomfort has disappeared, usually within $1/2$-1 minute, a second instillation is made. If this should again cause smarting, a further instillation is required. Thus the application of the anaesthetic agent may be used as a test of its own effect.

DEEPLY EMBEDDED FOREIGN BODY

Anaesthesia of the cornea for the removal of

Fig. 9

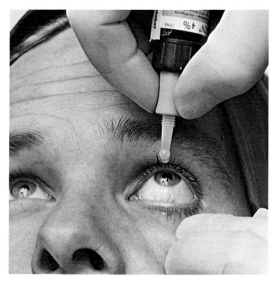

a *deeply embedded foreign body* generally requires repeated instillations, especially if it is situated in the area of the limbus, where the blood vessels – dilated because of irritation – rapidly remove the anaesthetic agent.

ANAESTHESIA OF THE CONJUNCTIVA

Anaesthesia of the conjunctiva requires frequent instillations repeated at short intervals, particularly if the conjunctiva is inflamed, whether postoperatively or because of infection. For instance as many as 20 instillations over a period of 5-10 minutes may be required for the removal of sutures.

Almost all operations on the eye commence with surface anaesthesia. Often this has to be augmented by further instillations during the course of the operation.

N.B. Preparations containing viscosity increasing agents such as methyl cellulose should be avoided for surgical interventions on the eye, since they could penetrate into the eyeball. Thus lignocaine 4 % topical solution should be used instead of the specially prepared eye drops.

Fig. 10

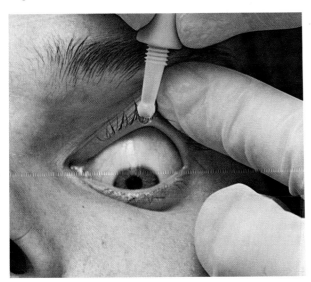

Infiltration Anaesthesia in Ophthalmology

Björn Wulfing

Infiltration anaesthesia is employed in ophthalmology for all operations on the eyelid and tearduct.

Anaesthesia of the Eyelid

The basic structure of the eyelid, the tarsal plate, limits the spread of the anaesthetic agent. Therefore it is necessary to inject both into the skin and the conjunctival aspects of the eyelid. However, this can be effected by only one injection. Here the procedure on the lower eyelid is demonstrated.

The needle (1.5 cm.) pierces the skin at the lower lateral margin of the tarsal plate and subcutaneous infiltration is performed with 2-3 ml. of lignocaine or prilocaine 0.5 % with vasoconstrictor (cf. fig. 16, p. 32).

The eyelid is everted, using the needle as a fulcrum, which is then thrust in until its point is prominent under the conjunctiva (fig. 11). Subconjunctival infiltration can then be carried out.

In this way the eyelid can be completely anaesthetized from a single insertion of the needle.

Fig. 11

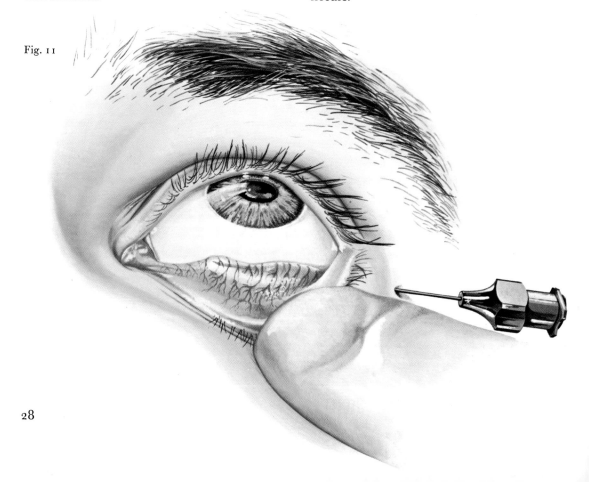

Anaesthesia of the Tearduct

SYRINGING OF THE TEARDUCT

For syinging of the tearduct instillation as previously described (cf. Surface Anaesthesia p. 26) is adequate. For passing a probe the duct is irrigated first with local anaesthetic solution.

OPERATIONS ON THE TEARSAC

The anaesthetic technique for operative procedures on the tearsac (dachryocystectomy, dachryocystorhinostomy) is demonstrated in figure 12.

The needle is inserted 0.5-1.0 cm. above the medial canthus in a backward and inward direction, until the resistance of the orbital septum is felt. Then 1 ml. of lignocaine or prilocaine 0.5 % with vasoconstrictor is injected.

The needle is withdrawn partially and then redirected more medially and somewhat backwards, towards the bone of the upper part of the fossa of the lacrimal sac, where 0.5 ml. is injected. The needle is removed and the injected area compressed with the thumb so that the anaesthetic solution is spread downwards around the sac.

The needle is inserted 1 cm. below and slightly medial to the medial canthus, and 0.5 ml. of a 0.5 % solution of lignocaine or prilocaine with vasoconstrictor is injected subcutaneously. The needle is then directed upwards and backwards towards the bone, with its tip underneath the medial palpebral ligament, where 0.5 ml. is injected. Again the injected area is compressed with the thumb so that the anaesthetic solution is spread around the lower part of the tearsac.

For dachryocystorhinostomy the nasal mucous membrane adjacent to the tearsac is also anaesthetized. This is performed via the nares either by direct submucous injection, by inserting a tamponade soaked in anaesthetic solution into the nose or by the use of a spray (cf. surface anaesthesia of the nose p. 37).

Fig. 12

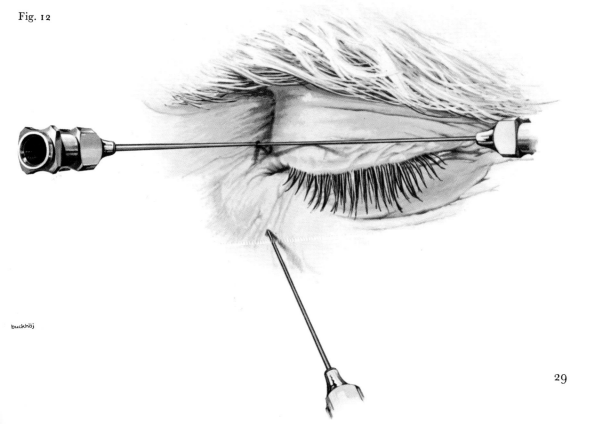

buckhöj

Conduction Anaesthesia for Intraocular Surgery

Björn Wulfing

Eyelid Paresis

Eyelid paresis can be achieved by anaesthetising the orbicularis oculi muscle according to the method of van Lint (fig. 13). This is necessary prior to all intraocular surgery, in order to prevent blepharospasm which can endanger the success of the operation.

The needle is inserted at right angles to the skin until the lower lateral angle of the inferior orbital margin is reached. Here, with the tip of the needle against the edge of the bone, 1 ml. of a 2 % solution of lignocaine or prilocaine with vasoconstrictor is injected.

The needle is then redirected and 2 ml. of the same solution are injected along the lateral margin of the orbit.

Still from the same point of insertion another 2 ml. of the solution are injected along the inferior orbital margin.

Fig. 13

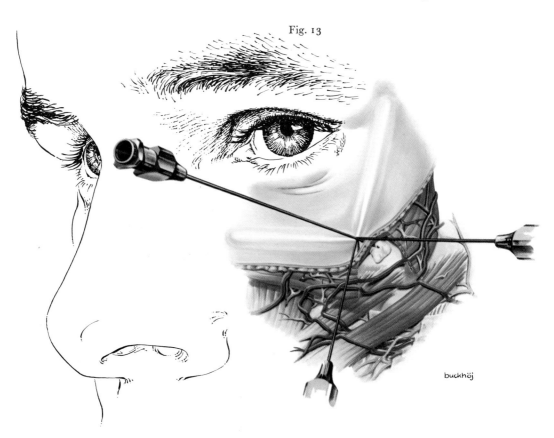

buckhöj

Fig. 14

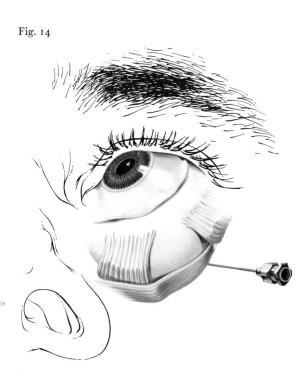

Retrobulbar Anaesthesia

ANATOMY

The *ciliary ganglion,* measuring 2-3 mm. in length, lies deep in the orbit just lateral to *the optic nerve* and medial to the lateral rectus muscle. Immediately behind the ganglion, the ophthalmic artery winds around the lateral side of *the optic nerve* and crossing above it passes forwards in a medial direction.

TECHNIQUE

The needle used should be exactly 3.5 cm. long or alternatively should bear a marker at this distance from its point, so as to reach the ciliary ganglion but at the same time avoiding the risk of puncturing the blood vessels in the apex of the orbit.

The injection is performed through the lower eyelid, at the lower lateral angle of the orbit. During the insertion of the needle the patient should look upwards and medially, which produces a contraction of the inferior oblique muscle and allows the needle to pass under it more easily (fig. 14). The anterior part of the eyeball is moved away from the needle, in order to gain better access to the ciliary ganglion (fig. 15).

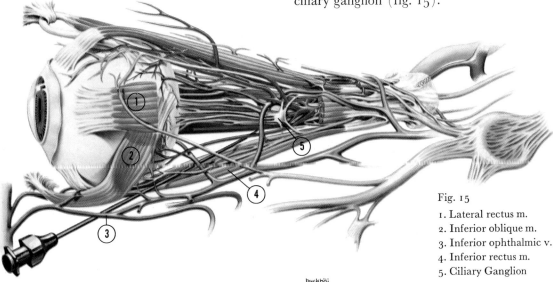

buckhöj

Fig. 15
1. Lateral rectus m.
2. Inferior oblique m.
3. Inferior ophthalmic v.
4. Inferior rectus m.
5. Ciliary Ganglion

The lower lateral angle of the orbit is palpated. The needle is inserted through the skin, where 0.5 ml. of a plain 2 % solution of lignocaine or prilocaine is injected. The needle is directed towards the apex of the orbit, i.e. backwards, inwards and upwards (fig. 17).

Slowly and while injecting simultaneously 0.5-1.0 ml. of solution (in order to displace any blood vessel along the path of the needle) the needle is inserted in its entire length or alternatively up to the marker, i.e. exactly 3.5 cm. (fig. 18). Careful aspiration is essential to exclude the possibility of an intravenous injection. Then 1.5-2 ml. of a plain 2 % solution of lignocaine or prilocaine are administered, taking 5-10 seconds over the injection. If complete akinesia is desired, the volume injected should be increased to 4 ml.

After removal of the needle, five minutes should be allowed to elapse before surgery is commenced.

NORMAL RESPONSE

The pupil dilates, and the intraocular pressure is reduced. Partial or total paralysis of the extrinsic muscles of the eye is achieved.

Retrobulbar anaesthesia always produces slight exophthalmos, directly proportional to the volume injected. The recommended volume of 1.5-2.0 ml. is adequate for the majority of intraocular procedures, but larger doses (at least 4 ml.) are recommended for enucleation, or for the photo- or electro-coagulation of the retina.

COMPLICATIONS

Retrobulbar haemotoma. This rarely occurs unless the needle is inserted for more than 3.5 cm. If a haematoma should form, it always does so within five minutes of the injection. In such a case the operation is deferred until the exophthalmos has regressed. If exophthalmos is marked a pressure dressing is applied.

PARALYSIS OF THE SUPERIOR RECTUS MUSCLE

Frequently the patient will still be able to move the eyeball upwards to a certain extent. Since this may be a disadvantage in intraocular surgery, retrobulbar anaesthesia may have to be augmented by anaesthesia of the superior rectus muscle.

The patient is asked to look downwards, and the upper eyelid is retracted. A 2 cm. long needle is inserted into Tenon's capsule (fascia bulbi) at the lateral edge of the superior rectus muscle and 1 ml. lignocaine or prilocaine 1.0 % with vasoconstrictor is injected into the belly of the muscle, posterior to the equator of the eyeball (fig. 19).

Fig. 16 (cf. p. 26)   Fig. 17

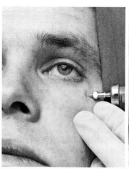 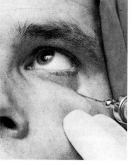

Fig. 18   Fig. 19

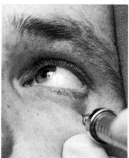 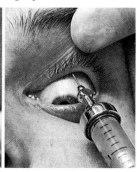

Anaesthesia for Ear, Nose and Throat Surgery

Tomas Gejrot

ANATOMY

The *auricle* is mainly innervated by *the great auricular nerve*. This nerve, a branch of the *cervical plexus*, becomes subcutaneous posterior to the mid-point of the sternocleidomastoid muscle *(punctum nervosum)* from which point it runs straight up towards the ear. Here it supplies the whole of the medial aspect of the auricle by a posterior branch and the lower and peripheral part of its lateral aspect by an anterior branch. The anterior-superior part of the lateral surface of the auricle is innervated by the *auriculo-temporal nerve* (from the *mandibular nerve,* the third branch of the trigeminal nerve), which runs up immediately in front of the external auditory canal. *The concha* is innervated by the *auricular branch of the vagus nerve,* which emerges through the tympano-mastoid fissure, immediately anterior to the mastoid process and right behind the external auditory meatus.

The *external auditory meatus* is innervated partly by the *auriculotemporal nerve* and partly by *the auricular branches of the vagus nerve.* The former gives off a *branch to the external auditory meatus* as it passes in front of the external auditory canal, which it enters at the junction between the cartilagenous and the bony parts of the external auditory meatus. It then supplies the skin of the upper, anterior and lower boundaries of the aural canal, along with the tympanic membrane. The auricular *branch of the vagus nerve* innervates the skin of the lower and posterior walls of the auditory canal.

The tympanic cavity obtains its sensory innervation through *the tympanic nerve,* a branch of the glossopharyngeal nerve, which enters the cavity through the canaliculus for the tympanic nerve and forms a plexus over the promontory.

Paracentesis

Two or three metered spray doses of lignocaine 10 % aerosol spray (20-30 mg.) are directed towards the upper wall of the auditory canal and are allowed to run down over the ear-drum (fig. 20). This reduces the discomfort which results from spraying the cold solution directly on to the drum. Paracentesis may be performed after 3-5 minutes.

INDICATIONS

This form of analgesia is used in conjunction with the treatment of otitis and otosalpingitis in patients of all age groups, with the exception of unsedated young children, who cannot be kept still. An absolute indication exists if the patient has recently taken fluids.

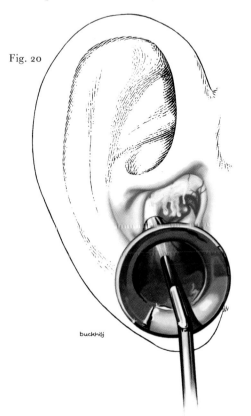

Fig. 20

buckhöj

Radical Mastoidectomy

TECHNIQUE

The great auricular nerve is blocked by the injection of 1-2 ml. of lignocaine solution into a number of sites over the mastoid process (fig. 21). The auricular branch is blocked by the injection of 2-3 ml. of lignocaine solution, part of it into the skin lining the floor of the auditory canal and the rest periosteally on the anterior part of the mastoid process (fig. 22). The auriculotemporal nerve is anaesthetized by the injection of 2 ml. into the junction between the bony and cartilagenous parts of the anterior wall of the auditory canal (tympanic branch) and partly by the infiltration of the skin and periosteum around the incicura terminalis over the auditory canal in front of the ear (fig. 24).

Should surface anaesthesia of the mucous membrane of the antrum, epitympanum or tympanum be required, 4-5 drops of 4 % lignocaine may be instilled.

DOSAGE

1-3 ml. of 0.5-1.0 % lignocaine with adrenaline in each injection, 10-15 ml. in all.

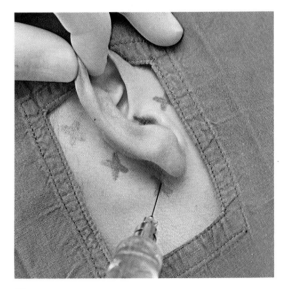

Fig. 21

INDICATIONS

Co-operative patients above the age of 15 years and when general anaesthesia is contra-indicated.

CONTRAINDICATIONS

Children under 15 years of age and nervous patients.

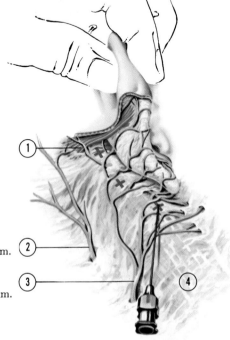

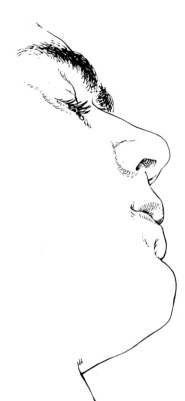

Fig. 22
1. Posterior auricularis m.
2. Lesser occipital n.
3. Great auricular n.
4. Sternocleidomastoid m.

34

Tympanotomy

The injection of 2 ml. lignocaine 2 % with adrenaline into the junction between the bony and cartilagenous parts of the anterior wall of the auditory canal is usually adequate (fig. 23) for anaesthesia of the auriculo-temporal nerve and its tympanic branch (fig. 24). Should the auditory canal be narrow or an endaural incision be necessary, infiltration anterior to the ear and the floor of the auditory canal must be performed, as for a radical mastoidectomy.

DOSAGE

2-5 ml. of lignocaine 2 % with adrenaline.

INDICATIONS

Local anaesthesia should be used when operations for otosclerosis are being performed, to permit simultaneous audiometry. If tympanotomy is being performed for some other reason, as, for example, an exploratory procedure, or if the patient is very anxious, general anaesthesia may be considered. Should the patient complain of nausea during the operation, this may be abolished by the intravenous injection of 1 % lignocaine in a dose of 1 mg./kg. body weight.

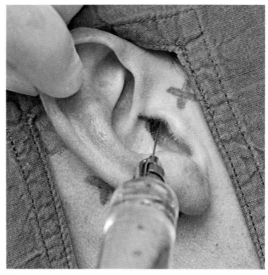

Fig. 23

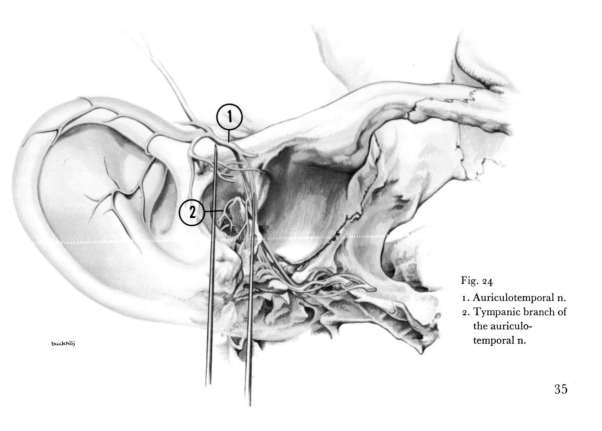

Fig. 24
1. Auriculotemporal n.
2. Tympanic branch of the auriculo-temporal n.

buckhöj

35

Operations on the Outer Nose and Septum

ANATOMY

Both the inner and outer aspects of the nose are innervated by the trigeminal nerve (see p. 58).

TECHNIQUE

The outer nose is anaesthetized with 5 to 8 ml. lignocaine, beginning at the tip. The infiltration is made subcutaneously, from the glabella down over the lateral aspects of the nose, during withdrawl of the needle to avoid undue distension of the tissues, and resultant change in the nasal contour. Alternatively, the skin can be penetrated at the glabella, and the needle passed downwards to the alae nasi. The needle is then not withdrawn completely, but angled medially. Usually about four anaesthetic tracks on each side will ensure good anaesthesia of the nasal walls.

The bases of the alae nasi are anaetshetized separately, together with the area down to the back of the nostrils, and the piriform aperture. From this point the region involved in a planned lateral osteotomy can be anaesthetized up to the level of the medial ligament of the canthus.

The mucoperichondrium of the nasal septum and the mucosa of the lateral walls of the nose are anaesthetized with 1–2 cm broad tampons, soaked in 4 % lignocaine with addition of 0,1 % adrenaline. The tampons should be left in situ for about 10 minutes. The membranous septum and the base of the columella are anaesthetized with 1 % lignocaine. The posterior aspect of the nasopharynx is lightly packed to absorb blood, and prevent secretions running down to the oropharynx during operation.

Another common and effective method of anaesthetizing the nasal septum is to inject lignocaine 0,5–1 % submucoperichondrially at the operation site. This method is best combined with anaesthesia of the nostrils effected by lignocaine tampons or lignocaine spray (10 mg./spray).

DOSAGE

Lignocaine 1 % 5–8 ml. for anaesthesia of the outer nose.

Lignocaine 0,5 (0,5–1 %) % 5–8 ml. for anaesthesia of each side of the nasal septum. Lignocaine 4 % with addition of 0,2 ml. 0,1 % adrenaline solution/ml. lignocaine solution. For nasal packing.

CONTRAINDICATIONS

Nervous adults and children. Fractures of the nose should generally be repaired under general anaesthesia.

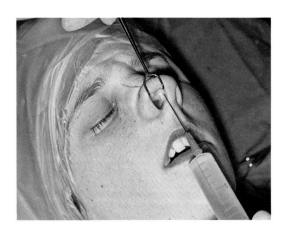
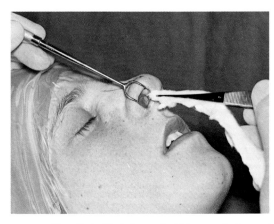

(Skoog Tord: Plastic Surgery. Stockholm 1974. Boston 1973)

Puncture of the Maxillary Sinus

ANATOMY

The posterior part of the lateral wall of the nasal cavity receives its nerve supply from the *posterior nasal branches* of *the maxillary nerve,* while the anterior part is supplied by branches from the *anterior ethmoidal nerve* (arising from the *ophthalmic nerve* the branches of which gain access to the nasal cavity through some of the anterior holes in the lamina cribrosa (fig. 25). (See also "The trigeminal nerve – an anatomical survey", p. 58).

TECHNIQUE

Should the conchae be swollen, a cotton wool swab soaked in a 4 % solution of lignocaine with adrenaline is inserted under the medial and inferior conchae for at least ten minutes. Surface anaesthesia of the site of puncture under the inferior concha may be induced with advantage using a 10 % lignocaine aerosol spray, which delivers a metered dose (10 mg. of lignocaine) with each pressing of the valve. This gives a slight stinging sensation in the nose for an instant. Puncture can be performed after 1-3 minutes.

DOSAGE

Pledgets of cotton wool (eye-swabs on sticks) are soaked in 4 % lignocaine with 2-3 drops (0.15 ml.) of 0.1 % adrenaline for every 5 ml. solution. Alternatively 1-3 spray doses of the 10 % lignocaine aerosol spray at the puncture-site under the inferior concha result in anaesthesia lasting half an hour.

CONTRAINDICATIONS

Children under 10 and particularly young ones under 5 years of age.

Fig. 25
1. Anterior ethmoidal n.
2. Lateral posterior superior nasal nn.
3. Pterygopalatine ganglion
4. Posterior inferior nasal branches

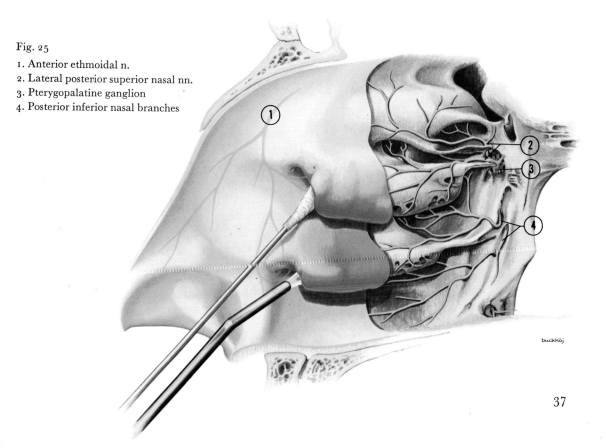

buckhöj

Caldwell-Luc Operation

ANATOMY

The *anterior superior alveolar rami* arise from the *infraorbital nerve,* and run down through fine bone canaliculi to join the *superior dental plexus,* which is formed by the mingling of the *posterior, medial and anterior superior alveolar rami,* and lies at the base of the alveolar process above the root apices (fig. 27). These branches of the *infraorbital nerve* supply the maxillary sinus and the adjacent area.

TECHNIQUE

Ten minutes before infiltration anaesthesia the mucous membrane of the gingiva is sprayed twice with 4 % lignocaine, with a 5 minute interval. The nasal cavity on the side to be operated is packed with ribbon gauze soaked in 4 % lignocaine. On the operating table the mucous membrane and periosteum above the premolars is infiltrated with 0.5-1 % lignocaine with vasoconstrictor (fig. 26, 27). When the maxillary sinus has been opened, further injections may be made into and under the mucous membrane.

DOSAGE

Approximately 1 ml. of lignocaine 4 %, followed by 8-10 ml. of lignocaine 0.5-1 % with adrenaline injected into the gingival mucous membrane and an additional 5-10 ml. around the mucous membrane of the sinus.

CONTRAINDICATIONS

Children under 15 years of age and nervous adults.

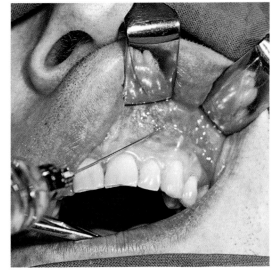

Fig. 26

Fig. 27

1. Anterior superior alveolar branches
2. Superior dental plexus
3. Branches to the teeth
4. Branches to the upper gum

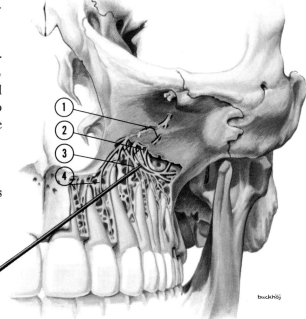

buckhöj

Laryngoscopy, Tracheoscopy and Bronchoscopy

ANATOMY

The larynx receives its nerve supply partly from the *superior laryngeal nerve* and partly from the *inferior laryngeal nerve,* both being branches of the *vagus nerve.* The *superior laryngeal nerve* arises from the *vagus nerve* immediately below its *inferior ganglion* and runs obliquely downwards and forwards, crossing from the lateral side the posterior part of the greater cornu of the hyoid bone and descending along the outside of the thyrohyoid membrane. Here the nerve gives off a small *external branch* to the crico-thyrohyoid membrane accompanied by the i.e. the *internal laryngeal nerve,* pierces the thyreohyoid membrane accompanied by the superior thyroid artery and vein, to supply the mucous membrane of the larynx down to the rima glottidis. In the piriform fossa this nerve forms a little fold of mucous membrane – the plica nervi laryngei. The *inferior laryngeal nerve,* which is the terminal branch of the *recurrent nerve,* supplies the laryngeal muscles (with the exception of the crico-thyroid muscle) as well as the mucous membrane of the larynx below the rima glottidis. The *trachea and bronchi* are supplied by branches of the *vagus nerve.*

TECHNIQUE

The throat – and, in edentulous patients, the gingiva also – is sprayed twice at five-minute intervals, using a 4 % solution of lignocaine or prilocaine. Then, the laryngeal aspect of the epiglottis and the larynx are anaesthetized, using a laryngeal syringe and a la-

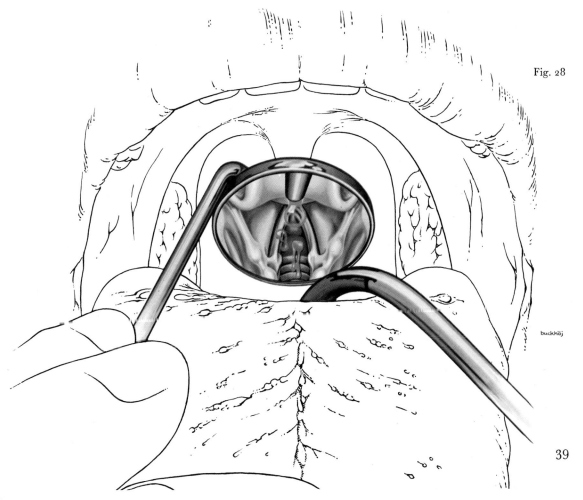

Fig. 28

buckhöj

39

ryngeal mirror (fig. 28). The local anaesthetic should always be administered during intonation, irrespective of the procedure. The anaesthetic solution should be allowed to run down the trachea – it should not be squirted down (fig. 29). This is repeated after five minutes. It is more comfortable for the patient if a laryngeal spray is used, but care must be taken to avoid overdosage.

If the patient still experiences discomfort or has an irritating cough, the trachea can be directly anaesthetized by the transtracheal injection of 1-2 ml. of 2 % lignocaine through the cricothyroid membrane.

As an alternative technique an aerosol spray of 10 % lignocaine may be employed for the whole procedure bearing in mind that each metered spray-dose provides exactly 10 mg. of lignocaine. In this way a more

efficient dispersal of the solution is achieved and onset of anaesthesia is more rapid. The average number of metered 10 mg. spray doses required are 3-5 for laryngoscopy and 5-10 for tracheoscopy and bronchoscopy respectively. Each metered dose should be given at approximately ½ minute intervals.

DOSAGE
0.5-1 ml. repeated at 3-5 minute intervals of of lignocaine 4 % solution (maximum total dose 5 ml.) or prilocaine 4 % solution (maximum total dose 10 ml.).

10 % lignocaine aerosol spray according to the above recommendations, not exceeding a total number of 20 sprays (200 mg.).

CONTRAINDICATIONS
Children under 15 years of age.

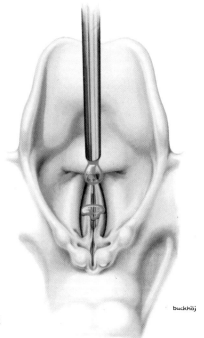
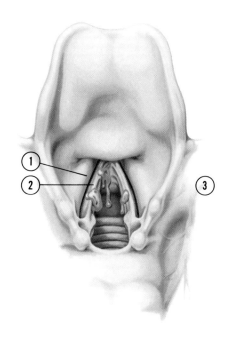

Fig. 29
1. Vestibular fold
2. Vocal fold
3. Superior laryngeal n.

buckhöj

Fibreoptic Bronchoscopy

TECHNIQUE

When using the transnasal approach, the larger nostril should be selected and sprayed three to four times with lignocaine 10 mg./ml. The patient is instructed to inhale, and this transports the local anaesthetic down to the level of the vocal cords.

On occasion, but rarely, it may be necessary also to spray the mouth and oro-pharynx.

The chosen nostril is lubricated with lignocaine gel to reduce friction.

The other nostril also is lightly anaesthetized, and a small catheter inserted, through which continous oxygen is given during the procedure. The fibreoptic bronchoscope is inserted to the level of the epiglottis and laryngeal introitus, and, here, 3–4 aliquots of 0,5-1,0 ml. lignocaine (10 mg./ml.) are injected with a syringe down the scope's lumen. After a few minutes' pause, the scope is passed into the trachea. During the progression of the bronchoscope, further aliquots of 0,5–1,0 ml. lignocaine (10 mg./ml.) are given as necessary.

Total dosage should not exceed 300 mg. lignocaine.

Ollman et al, (1975) use a specially adapted polyvinyl catheter, which is passed down the bronchoscope lumen.

The local anaesthesia is given by an aerosol spray attached to the catheter. Each press gives a spray containing 10 mg. lignocaine. This is a good method, which allows acurate control of the supplementary lignocaine dosage.

Contraindications lignocaine allergy. Note that patients with chronic bronchitis usually need higher dosages of local anaesthetic.

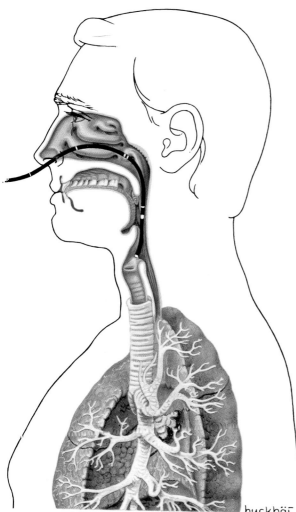

buckhöj

Tonsillectomy

ANATOMY

The area of the tonsils is innervated by the *tonsillar branches of the glossopharyngeal nerve,* the trunk of which runs along the stylopharyngeal muscle (Fig. 30).

TECHNIQUE

With the patient lying down, surface anaesthesia of the throat, the base of the tongue, the anterior and posterior palatal arches is first induced by spraying with 4 % lignocaine, repeated after an interval of five minutes. The patient is then positioned in the chair, and infiltration anaesthesia is carried out using a tonsil syringe. The first injection is placed under the mucous membrane of the posterior palatal arch, so as not to get in the way of further injections (fig. 30). After this, the anterior palatal arch is injected, as well as the remaining superficial peritonsillar tissue and the floor of the mouth. The tongue is depressed by means of a spatula, so that the base of the tongue and the tonsillar attachment can be infiltrated (fig. 31). The tonsil can be drawn medially using a pair of tonsil forceps, to facilitate injection into the tonsillar plexus.

DOSAGE

Lignocaine 4 % or prilocaine 4 % for surface anaesthesia: approximately 1 ml. in all. Lignocaine 0.5 % (adrenaline 1:200.000) or prilocaine 0.5 % (adrenaline 1:250.000) 20-30 ml. – i.e. 10-15 ml. for each side.

CONTRAINDICATIONS

Children under 15 years of age, as well as anxious and uncooperative adults. Patients desiring general anaesthesia should be allowed their choice.

Fig. 30

1. Stylopharyngeal m.
2. Palatine tonsil
3. Tonsillar branches
4. Glossopharyngeal n.

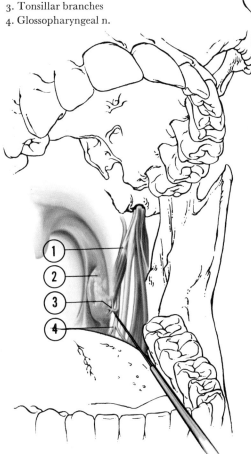

Fig. 31

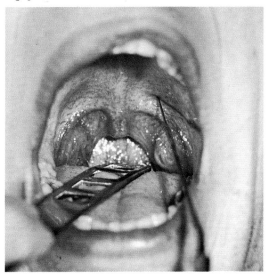

Local Anaesthesia for Thyroid Surgery

Viktor von Bahr

ANATOMY

The area of operation derives its most important nerve supply from superficial branches of the *cervical plexus*. These may be blocked easily at the mid-point of the posterior margin of the sternocleidomastoid muscle. The external jugular vein crosses the edge of the muscle at approximately this level (fig. 32).

Sensory nerves also accompany the superior thyroid artery to the superior pole of the thyroid gland.

TECHNIQUE

Before the operation, the patient should be well sedated. Further sedation may be required during the course of the operation.

Prilocaine 0.5 % with adrenaline 1:250.000 is used as the anaesthetic solution. Should the minimal quantities of adrenaline contained in this solution be considered undesirable or even contraindicated, as in patients with thyrotoxicosis, fully adequate anaesthesia may be obtained using the *plain* solution of 0.5 % prilocaine. However, in this case the duration of anaesthesia will be shorter and a further infiltration may become necessary should the operation be prolonged. As a rule, general anaesthesia frequently combined with local infiltration is preferable in these patients provided a trained anaesthetist is available.

The patient lies in the supine position. When the right side is being injected, the head is turned slightly to the left, and vice

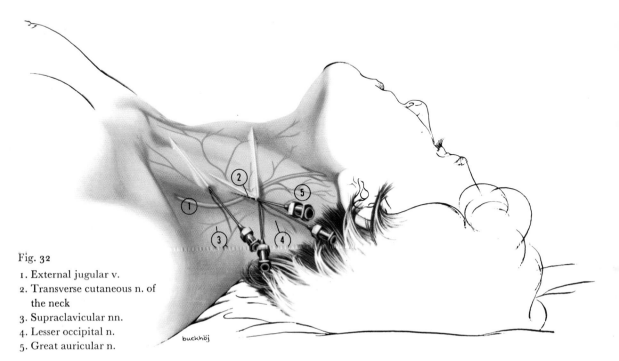

Fig. 32
1. External jugular v.
2. Transverse cutaneous n. of the neck
3. Supraclavicular nn.
4. Lesser occipital n.
5. Great auricular n.

buckhöj

43

versa. Using a fine gauge needle, two skin weals are raised, on either side of the neck in the middle of the posterior margin of the sternocleidomastoid muscle (fig. 32). From each of these weals, using a somewhat wider bore needle, 10-15 ml. of anaesthetic solution are injected on each side, subcutaneously and under the superficial fascia. In this way the superficial branches of the cervical plexus are blocked.

The dissection will be facilitated and bleeding reduced if the region of the proposed skin flaps between the jugular notch and the upper border of the larynx is infiltrated through the skin weals, using a long needle.

While it is possible to block pre-operatively the pain-transmitting fibres which accompany the superior thyroid artery, this is easier once the anterior surface of the thyroid gland has been exposed (fig. 33). To do this 1 or 2 ml. of solution are injected above its superior pole (fig. 34). Should traction on the gland cause discomfort a few millilitres may also be injected under the capsule of the thyroid gland (fig. 33, 34). However, this injection should not be given too far posteriorly, lest the recurrent nerve be blocked and the possibility of checking vocal chord activity during the operation be lost.

DOSAGE

70-80 ml. of 0.5 % prilocaine with adrenaline are usually required. If a vasoconstrictor is omitted, a further 30 ml. of solution may be required later on during the course of the operation.

INDICATIONS

Simple thyroidectomy in normal patients. Local anaesthesia in combination with heavy sedation is a relatively satisfactory technique for thyroid surgery. It may be considered an advantage that the activity of the vocal chords can be checked during the operation.

CONTRAINDICATIONS

This technique is not suitable for nervous patients, particularly those suffering from thyrotoxicosis, or for children.

COMPLICATIONS

There are no special risks associated with this technique, apart from that of blocking the recurrent laryngeal nerve, as mentioned above. Intravascular administration must, of course, be avoided by repeated aspiration.

Fig. 33

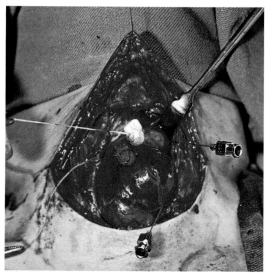

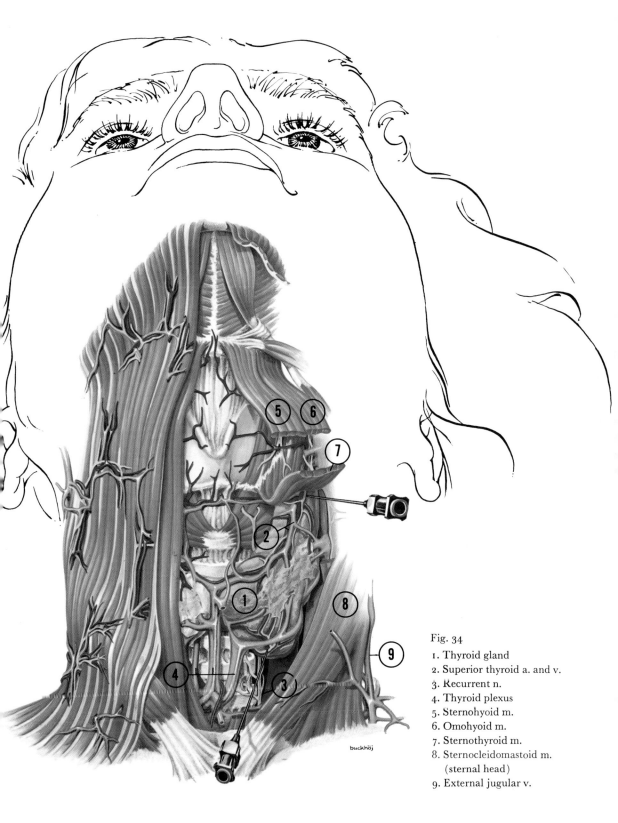

Fig. 34

1. Thyroid gland
2. Superior thyroid a. and v.
3. Recurrent n.
4. Thyroid plexus
5. Sternohyoid m.
6. Omohyoid m.
7. Sternothyroid m.
8. Sternocleidomastoid m.
   (sternal head)
9. External jugular v.

buckhöj

45

Infiltration of a Fracture Haematoma

EJNAR ERIKSSON

A spread of local anaesthetic solution both to the nerve fibres which supply the soft tissue around the fracture and to those which supply bone and periosteum may be obtained by injection into the haematoma around the fracture.

TECHNIQUE

The site of the fracture is palpated and the fracture haematoma is punctured. The correct position of the needle is verified by positive aspiration of blood into the syringe (fig. 35). The local anaesthetic solution without a vasoconstrictor is injected *slowly*. Rapid injection is very painful. After about five minutes the fracture can be reduced under relatively good anaesthesia. However, the anasthesia obtained is not comparable with that produced by conduction anaesthesia of the corresponding nerves (in the case of the upper extremity e.g. a brachial plexus block, pp. 79, 82 or intravenous regional anaesthesia, p. 47).

DOSAGE

10-15 ml. of prilocaine 1 or 2 % without vasoconstrictor.

10 ml. of lignocaine 2 % or 10-15 ml. of lignocaine 1 % without vasoconstrictor.

INDICATIONS

This method should never be recommended for routine use, since satisfactory anaesthesia can seldom be obtained. It may be indicated, when a limited number of doctors have to deal with mass casualties.

CONTRAINDICATIONS

This technique is absolutely contraindicated, when the skin is dirty or when other circumstances prevent an aseptic technique, because of the obvious risk of infecting a closed fracture.

N.B. There is also the risk of rapid absorption.

Fig. 35

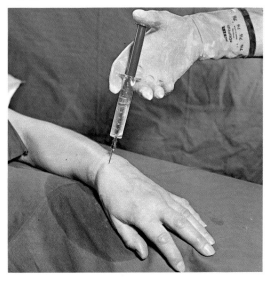

Intravenous Regional Anaesthesia

Anne-Marie Thorn-Alquist

The injection of a local anaesthetic into a vein in an extremity isolated from the circulation by means of a tourniquet was first described by Bier in 1908. However, this method did not come into widespread use until the recent introduction of powerful local anaesthetic agents of very low toxicity. (Holmes 1963, Bell et al. 1963, Adams et al. 1964, Merrifield & Carter 1965, Eriksson et al. 1966 among other workers).

Fig. 36

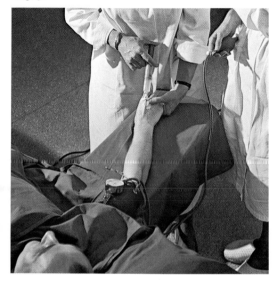

TECHNIQUE

A blood pressure cuff or pneumatic tourniquet is applied to the limb proximal to the site of operation and an indwelling needle such as the Gordh or better still, a plastic intravenous canula, is inserted into a peripheral vein. If a bloodless field is required by the surgeon, this may be obtained by the use of an Esmarch bandage. Otherwise the limb is elevated for a few minutes to decrease the amount of blood contained in it. The blood pressure cuff is inflated to a pressure of at least 50 mm. and usually 100-150 mm. Hg above the systolic pressure. The pressure required depends upon the size of the muscle mass to be compressed. It is clear that a stout muscular leg needs a higher pressure to occlude the arterial blood flow than a slender arm. Then the local anaesthetic solution is injected as a single dose through the indwelling needle, which may then be removed (fig. 36). Satisfactory analgesia and muscular relaxation are obtained after 10-15 minutes. When the operation is completed, the cuff is deflated. This, however, should not be done until at least 15 minutes have elapsed after the completion of the injection, because of the increased risk of toxic reaction. On return of the normal circulation the effect of the local anaesthetic rapidly disappears – usually within 2-5 minutes. Should it be desirable to release the blood pressure cuff before the end of the operation in order to secure any bleeding points, only a few minutes adequate analgesia can be expected, unless a suplementary dose of local anaesthetic solution is given. The pressure of the cuff usually becomes uncomfortable for the patient after 30-40 minutes. This discomfort may be eliminated by applying another cuff distal to the original one round an anaesthetized area. This is then inflated before the pressure in the original cuff is released.

CONTINUOUS TECHNIQUE

Anaesthesia is induced as described above. However, the intravenous needle is not removed after injecting the local solution but remains in situ until the operation is completed. The cuff may now be deflated whenever desired and as surgery is continued the cuff is re-inflated and anaesthesia supplemented by the injection of half the original dose through the indwelling needle (Brown and Weissman 1966).

DOSAGE

Lignocaine 0.5 %, procaine 0.5%, mepivacaine 0.5 % or prilocaine 0.5 .% The last named is the most suitable, since its sytemic toxicity is lowest. On no account must a vasoconstrictor be contained in the anaesthetic solution.

The quantity used depends on the volume of the limb involved. For the upper limb, when the cuff is applied around the middle part of the upper arm, 2-3 mg./kg body weight is a suitable dose for an adult of 70 kg. This is equivalent to approximately 40 ml. of a 0.5 % solution. For the lower limb, however, with the cuff in the mid-thigh position, a dose of 5-6 mg./kg body weight may be required equivalent to a volume of 60-80 ml. When such high doses are needed, prilocaine is recommended because of its low toxicity. In order to reduce the dose necessary for a leg the injection may be given between two cuffs. Significantly smaller quantities are required, yet anaesthesia is induced peripheral to the lower cuff.

INDICATIONS

This technique is remarkably simple and the method is well suited for operations particularly on the forearm and hand. It may also be used for surgery of the foot, and of the leg below the knee. The duration is limited by the time it is considered safe to occlude the circulation – 1 1/2 hours at the most. The continuous technique as described may be used for surgery of longer duration, since the cuff may be deflated at regular intervals. The rapid termination of anaesthesia after the cuff is deflated renders possible the assessment of nerve and tendon function immediately after the operation. Intravenous regional anaesthesia has been used successfully for many forms of surgery, such as the reduction of fractures (in which case care must be observed that the blood pressure cuff is not inflated with the muscles contracted), surgery of tendons, incisions and the suturing of wounds. It could well be suitable for amputations especially for mass casualties, since most of the local anaesthetic solution would be removed together with the limb.

CONTRAINDICATIONS

This method is less suitable for psychologically unstable patients, who would require heavy sedation and for patients with peripheral vascular or neurological disease. It should not be considered for patients with a history of oversensitivity to local anaesthetic agents.

COMPLICATIONS

Risk of toxic reactions is present when the cuff is deflated and the local anaesthetic agent released into the circulation. The patient should therefore be carefully observed during and after the release of the cuff. Some workers consider that intermittent release, deflating the tourniquet for only 5-10 seconds at a time, increases the margin of safety. Should symptoms of toxic reactions appear in spite of all precautions the scheme of treatment described on p. 16-17 should be instituted. Resuscitation equipment should always be immediately available (cf. p. 14).

Intraosseous Anaesthesia

ANNE-MARIE THORN-ALQUIST

The basic mechanism of intraosseous anaesthesia is a filling of the vascular bed by means of an injection of local anaesthetic solution into the bone marrow of an extremity which is isolated from the systemic circulation by a tourniquet (Orlov 1960, Ochotskij 1961).

TECHNIQUE

A blood pressure cuff is fixed to the limb, proximal to the site of the operation. The extremity is rendered ischaemic as for regional i.v. anaesthesia.

At the appropriate site (e.g. calcaneus) a bone-needle is inserted into the bone marrow (fig. 37). The local anaesthetic solution is injected through this needle very slowly and gently, especially at first, in order to minimize the patient's discomfort. Strict asepsis is essential.

In all other respects, i.e. dosage, latency period, duration, indications and contraindications, intraosseous anasthesia resembles intravenous regional anaesthesia (c.f. p. 47).

N.B. The risk of toxic reactions is the same as with intravenous regional anaesthesia and the same safety precautions should be taken.

Fig. 37

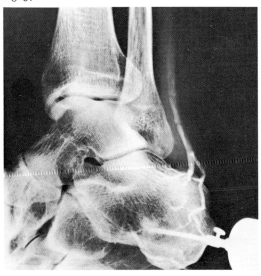

Digital Nerve Block

EJNAR ERIKSSON

ANATOMY

Each digit is supplied by four nerve branches – two dorsal and two palmar (or plantar respectively) which run forward along the respective edge of the digit (fig. 38).

TECHNIQUE

The nerves of the fingers and toes are easily blocked at the base of the respective digit. About 0.5-0.1 ml. is infiltrated into the approximate course of each nerve. No attempt is made to elicit paraesthesia. It is adequate to infiltrate superficially and deeply on both sides of the finger. Excessive volumes of local anaesthetic solution should be avoided, since the mechanical pressure of the solution in this tight area may obstruct the blood supply to the digit. Some orthopaedic surgeons (Moberg 1964) dislike this form of anaesthesia, because of this risk of mechanically in-duced ischaemia. However, at the Karolinska Hospital, Stockholm, this simple method has been used as a routine for about twenty years, without any undesirable sequelae.

DOSAGE

2-4 ml. lignocaine 1 % (-2 %) or prilocaine 1 % (-2 %). The use of a vasoconstrictor should be avoided (cf. pp. 16, 24).

INDICATIONS

Simple operations on the fingers or toes.

CONTRAINDICATIONS

In the case of more extensive injuries it is often advisable to choose a more proximal site for the block (wristblock, p. 90, nerve block at the elbow, p. 86, or brachial plexus block, pp. 79, 82, respectively).

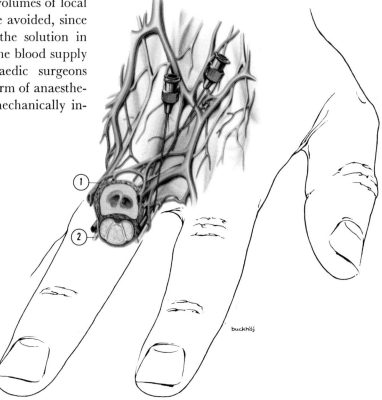

Fig. 38
1. Proper dorsal digital n.
2. Proper palmar digital n.

Infiltration Anaesthesia for Caesarian Section

Torsten Gordh

ANATOMY

The abdominal wall receives its nerve supply from the six lower intercostal nerves and inferiorly from the lumbar nerves. These nerves give off cutaneous branches just lateral to the midline.

TECHNIQUE

The technique is simple (fig. 39). Infiltration anaesthesia between the symphysis pubis to a point somewhat above the umbilicus is usually adequate. A long weal of local anaesthetic is raised about two fingers breadth on either side of the linea alba, reaching from the symphysis pubis to a point 5 cm. above the umbilicus. Using a 10 cm. needle the abdominal wall is infiltrated. The needle should always be parallel to the surface of the skin. The local anaesthetic agent is injected both during insertion and withdrawal of the needle until a raised weal has been produced on both sides of the linea alba. Care must be taken not to go through the peritoneum and pierce the uterus, since the abdominal wall is extremely thin in a patient at term. Naturally, even when local anaesthesia is employed oxygen must be given to the mother while the uterus is being opened and until the umbilical cord is tied.

DOSAGE

Up to 100 ml. of 0.25 % lignocaine with adrenaline 1:200.000 are usually adequate.

INDICATIONS

It is important to know that caesarian section *can* be carried out by infiltration anaesthesia alone. This should be borne in mind particularly in patients in poor general condition and in certain extreme situations such as severely impaired lung function, poliomyelitis, myasthenia gravis and in patients under respirator treatment. In such patients one may hesitate to employ general anaesthesia and spinal anaesthesia is contraindicated.

Local anaesthesia, when used alone, can be distressing to the patient. Moreover, it is difficult to avoid completely pain reflexes caused by traction on the uterus and manipulations of the intestines and the mesentery. However, local anaesthesia, as described above, is an excellent complement to general anaesthesia. The incision and suturing of the skin will be painless, a shallower plane of anaesthesia may be maintained and the patient will wake up more quickly than otherwise would be the case.

Fig. 39

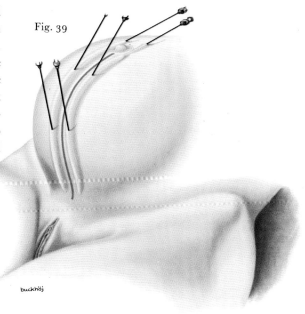

buckhöj

Local Anaesthesia for Inguinal Herniorrhaphy

Viktor von Bahr

ANATOMY

The inguinal area is supplied by three nerves, *the iliohypogastric, the ilioinguinal and the genitofemoral nerve* (fig. 40) all of which come from the lumbar plexus. The *iliohypogastric nerve* (L 1) gives off an anterior cutaneous branch which runs in a ventrocaudal direction, lying between the transversus and internal oblique muscles. It reaches the lower part of the anterior abdominal wall two fingers' breadth medial to the anterior superior iliac spine to supply the skin immediately above the inguinal ligament. The *ilioinguinal nerve* (L 1) runs parallel to but slightly below the iliohypogastric nerve. This nerve emerges through the superficial inguinal ring and gives off branches to the adjacent skin and to the scrotum (labia majora). The *genitofemoral nerve* (L 1 and L 2) divides up on the anterior aspect of the major psoas muscle, just above the inguinal ligament, into *a genital and a femoral branch.* The former follows the spermatic cord supplying the cremaster muscle and the skin of the scrotum (labia majora), while the latter traverses the lacuna vasorum on the lateral side of the external iliac artery to supply the skin over the upper part of the femoral triangle.

Autonomic fibres accompany the spermatic cord to the testis.

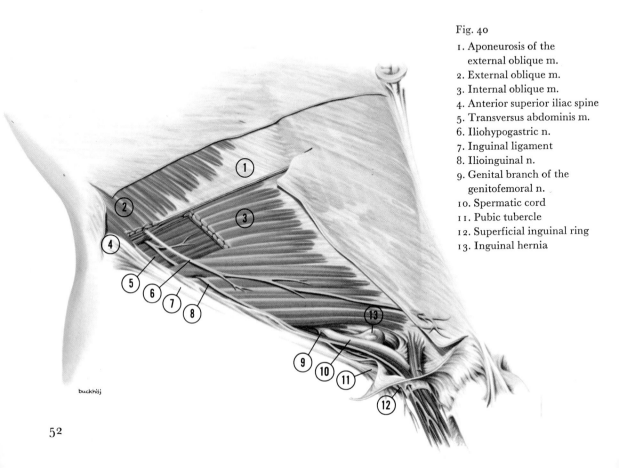

Fig. 40

1. Aponeurosis of the external oblique m.
2. External oblique m.
3. Internal oblique m.
4. Anterior superior iliac spine
5. Transversus abdominis m.
6. Iliohypogastric n.
7. Inguinal ligament
8. Ilioinguinal n.
9. Genital branch of the genitofemoral n.
10. Spermatic cord
11. Pubic tubercle
12. Superficial inguinal ring
13. Inguinal hernia

buckhöj

Prilocaine 0.5 % with adrenaline is used as the local anaesthetic. From a point two fingers' breadth medial to the anterior superior iliac spine the muscles in front of the pelvic bone are infiltrated (fig. 42), using 15-20 ml. of solution. From the same point of injection a further 15-20 ml. are injected under the aponeurosis of the external oblique muscle; part of this is injected directly caudal to the site of injection, the rest in a medio-caudal direction (fig. 41). In each case, the injection is performed immediately after penetrating the aponeurosis of the external oblique muscle. This can easily be felt if a needle with a short bevelled point is used. Still from the same point, a subcutaneous injection is performed in a lateral direction towards the inguinal fold and medio-caudally as far as the midline (fig. 41). A total of 10-30 ml. of solution will be used for this, the amount required depending upon the depth of the layer of fat.

From a second point immediately proximal to the pubic tubercle, 5-10 ml. of solution are injected extraperitoneally, along the superior margin of the pubic bone (fig. 41). From the same point approximately 5 ml. are injected within the aponeurosis of the external oblique muscle and about 5 cm. cranially. Subcutaneously injections are made in a fanwise manner, laterally as far as the inguinal fold and medio-cranially as far as the mid-line.

In the case of a reducible hernia, an injection can also be made along the spermatic cord at the superficial inguinal ring. However, in the author's experience, it is preferable to postpone this injection until the inguinal canal has been opened, thereby elimi-

Fig. 41

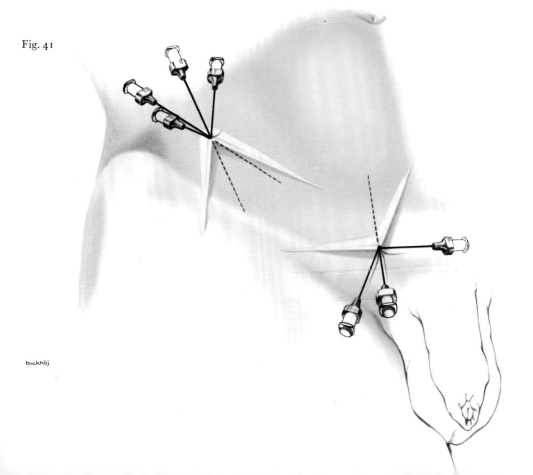

buckhöj

nating the risk of perforating the contents of the hernial sac or producing a haematoma in the spermatic cord. As usual, frequent aspiration tests are necessary to avoid intravascular injection. This is of special importance near the iliac vessels.

When an indirect inguinal hernia is being operated upon a few ml. of solution are injected from inside the hernial neck extraperitoneally, both medially and laterally, once the hernial sac has been opened and the hernia reduced (fig. 43). This facilitates dissection and renders manipulation of the hernial sac completely painless. If the hernia cannot be reduced without pain, a corresponding injection is performed from the outside around the neck of the hernia.

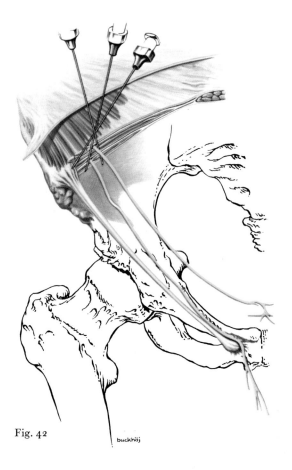

DOSAGE

The total amount required varies between 60 and 90 ml. of the 0.5 % solution of prilocaine with adrenaline 1:250.000.

INDICATIONS

Local infiltration anaesthesia carries the least risk and is especially indicated for patients who are bad risks for either general or spinal anaesthesia. Local infiltration anaesthesia may also be used in strangulated herniae with intestinal obstruction. In these patients there is a greater risk of vomiting and unless facilities for intubation anaesthesia with a cuffed endotracheal tube are available it is an advantage if the reflexes are intact in such patients.

CONTRAINDICATIONS

This method is hardly suitable for children or anxious patients. It is relatively contraindicated in very fat individuals with irreducible herniae as the landmarks may be difficult to palpate. These risks must be judged in relation to the possible hazards associated with general anaesthesia in such patients.

Fig. 42

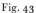

Fig. 43

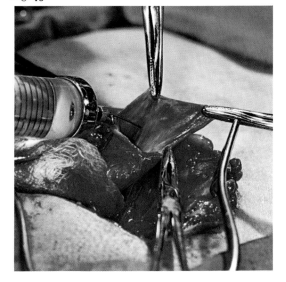

Local Anaesthesia of the Urethra

EJNAR ERIKSSON

EJNAR ERIKSSON

ANATOMY

Local anaesthetic agents deposited in the urethra can diffuse through its mucous membrane and so anaesthetize the nerve plexus which lies superficially under the mucosa.

TECHNIQUE

Local anaesthetic agents may be instilled into the urethra in the form of an aqueous solution or as a gel. The practical advantages of the gel are that the urethra is lubricated simultaneously, which facilitates the ensuing instrumentation and that the gel remains longer in contact with the mucous membrane which may improve the penetration of the local anaesthetic into the mucosa.

On the other hand, these advantages are outweighed by the fact that a few patients may have a bulbo-cavernous connection. Thus, if an injection into the urethra is performed under pressure, the thin mucous membrane may be ruptured, and the substance injected may enter the bloodstream (fig. 45, 46). Therefore local anaesthesia of the urethra should be induced with an agent of the lowest possible toxicity, and one may even consider the use of aqueous solutions since an intravenous injection of the gel (methylcellulose) may itself cause a serious reaction. The inferior anaesthetic effect of aqueous solutions is an argument against their use.

The anaesthetic agent is instilled slowly and under low pressure from a syringe or the

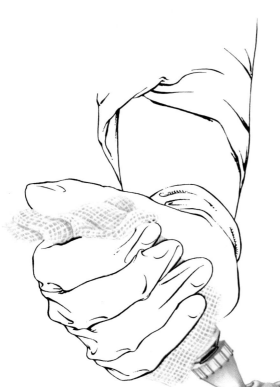

Fig. 44

55

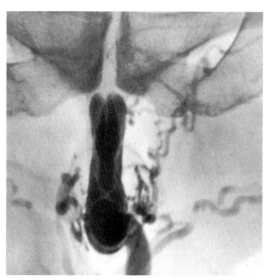

Fig. 45*

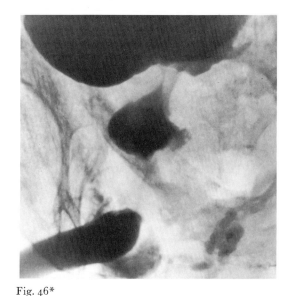

Fig. 46*

tube of gel, both being equipped with a cone (fig. 44). The penile part of the urethra should first be filled, using 10 ml. of solution or about one half of the tube. The patient is then asked to strain as when passing urine, whilst the rest of the solution or the gel is injected. Thus the injection is performed while the patient relaxes the inner sphincter and a certain amount of the anaesthetic agent reaches the prostatic portion of the urethra and the bladder neck. This is especially important since this is often the most sensitive site when a catheter or other instrument is being inserted. Following the injection a penile clamp is applied (fig. 47). In anaesthesia of the urethra in women, the major labia are held together so that the anaesthetic agent does not run out immediately. Anaesthesia of the mucous membrane is obtained within 4-5 minutes.

DOSAGE

Gel: 15-20 ml. prilocaine gel or lignocaine gel 2 %. (Aqueous solution: 15-20 ml. prilocaine or lignocaine 2 %).

* Reproduced by permission from N. P. G. Edling, M.D.

INDICATIONS

Catheterization, cystoscopy, passing of sounds, urethrocystography.

CONTRAINDICATIONS

The existence of a bulbocavernous reflux, known from X-ray examination (urethrocystography) since in this case there is a risk of a considerable amount of the anaesthetic being injected intravenously. Active bleeding may indicate open veins. Therefore the toxicity of the local anaesthetic agent employed is of the greatest importance.

Fig. 47

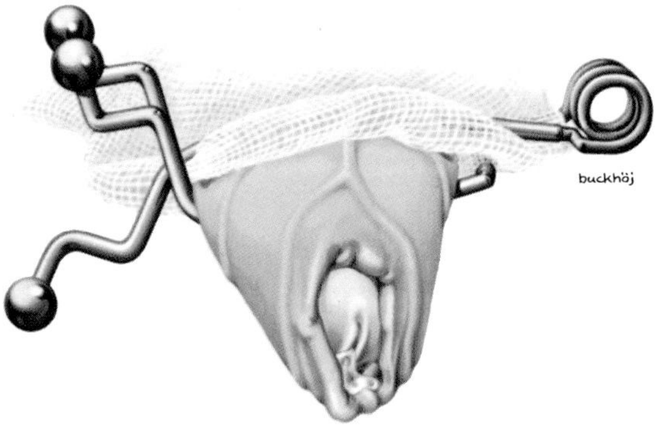

56

Surface Anaesthesia
of the Perineum
in Childbirth

Sören Englesson

Many countries lack an adequate obstetric and anaesthetic service and doctors with specialist qualifications cannot possibly be present at each delivery. Therefore, in Sweden, midwives are permitted to give certain forms of anaesthesia for the crowning of the head. However, their experience and training in the treatment of anaesthetic complications is very limited and there are constant efforts to find simpler and less dangerous methods.

Fig. 48

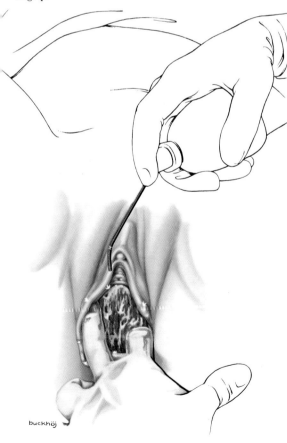

buckhöj

Surface anaesthesia of the mucous membranes offers an alternative, at least to a certain extent (Bergman & Malmström 1961).

TECHNIQUE

The local anaesthetic agent used is lignocaine 10 % in an aerosol container with a metered valve which automatically delivers a dose of 10 mg. lignocaine base per spray dose. Lignocaine is sprayed over the vulva and the vaginal introitus and on to the surface of minor lacerations (fig. 48).

The drug is administered during four phases of delivery:
1. When the foetal head begins to press against the floor of the pelvis.
2. When the perineum begins to bulge.
3. During crowning of the head.
4. After delivery, for repair of lacerations of the mucous membrane.

DOSAGE

The average number of spray doses administered at each stage is 10-15. Naturally the dosage has to be adjusted to the individual requirements. However, a total of 40 spray doses should not be exceeded, unless the delivery progresses very slowly (e.g. primiparae).

Estimations of the serum concentrations in maternal and foetal blood demonstrated the safety of this procedure (Bergman & Malmström 1963).

INDICATIONS

Deliveries in situations where other, more effective methods of analgesia are not available and as a supplement to other forms of analgesia and anaesthesia.

CONTRAINDICATIONS

There are no direct contraindications. However, should the method prove unsatisfactory the mother should be reassured that other more effective methods are available.

The Trigeminal Nerve-Anatomical Survey

Ture Petrén

The *trigeminal nerve* is a mixed nerve, which is made up of a large sensory part – *the portio major,* and a smaller motor part – *the portio minor.* The former has a large half-moon shaped ganglion – *ganglion semilunare* *(Gasseri)* or *trigeminal ganglion,* which fills the trigeminal impression in the floor of the middle cranial fossa. From the trigeminal ganglion arise the three large divisions of the nerve: *the ophthalmic nerve, the maxillary nerve* and *the mandibular nerve* (fig. 49).

THE OPHTHALMIC NERVE

The ophthalmic nerve is purely sensory. It enters the orbit through the superior orbital fissure, where it divides into three branches, namely: 1) *the lacrimal nerve,* which supplies branches to the conjunctiva and a small area of skin beside the lateral canthus of the eye and to the lacrimal gland; 2) the *nasociliary nerve* which runs medially, innervating the mucous membrane lining

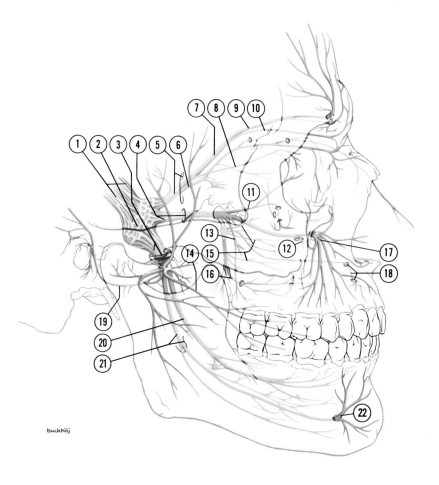

Fig. 49

1. Trigeminal n.
2. Gasserian ganglion
3. Mandibular n. and foramen ovale
4. Maxillary n. and foramen rotundum
5. Ophthalmic n. and superior orbital fissure
6. Nasociliary n.
7. Frontal n.
8. Lacrimal n.
9. Supraorbital n.
10. Supratrochlear n.
11. Zygomatic n.
12. Anterior superior alveolar branches
13. Posterior superior alveolar branches
14. Buccal n.
15. Posterior nasal branches
16. Greater palatine n.
17. Infraorbital n.
18. Nasopalatine n.
19. Auriculotemporal n.
20. Lingual n.
21. Inferior alveolar n.
22. Mental n.

the superior anterior part of the nasal cavity, along with the skin covering the upper part of the nose and that adjacent to the medial canthus of the eye; 3) *the frontal nerve,* which runs forward right under the roof of the orbit and divides into the *supraorbital* and *supratrochlear nerves* which innervate the skin of the upper eyelid and forehead, right up to the scalp (fig. 49, 50).

THE MAXILLARY NERVE

The maxillary nerve is entirely sensory. It passes through the foramen rotundum and enters the pterygopalatine fossa where it gives off its branches (fig. 49), of which the following are named here: 1) *the zygomatic nerve* which enters the orbit through the in-

ferior orbital fissure to course along the lateral wall of the orbit and ends by dividing into two branches which supply the skin of the anterior part of the temple and that adjacent to the lateral corner of the eye (fig. 50) 2) *the posterior nasal branches* supplying the mucous membrane lining the posterior inferior part of the nasal cavity. One of these branches, *the nasopalatine nerve* runs forwards and downwards along the nasal septum to the incisive foramen, through which it supplies branches to the anterior part of the hard palate and the adjacent area of gum; 3) *the greater palatine nerve* which reaches the hard palate through the greater palatine foramen to supply the mucous membrane of the hard palate and the palatal as-

Fig. 50

1. Supraorbital n.	8. Lateral branch of the frontal n.
2. Frontal n.	
3. Lacrimal n.	9. Medial branch of the frontal n.
4. Nasociliary n.	
5. Maxillary n.	10. Supratrochlear n.
6. Zygomatic n.	11. Infratrochlear n.
7. Infraorbital n.	12. Nasopalatine n.

Fig. 51

1. Posterior superior alveolar branches	4. Foramen rotundum
	5. Greater palatine n.
2. Infraorbital n.	6. Nasopalatine n.
3. Maxillary n.	

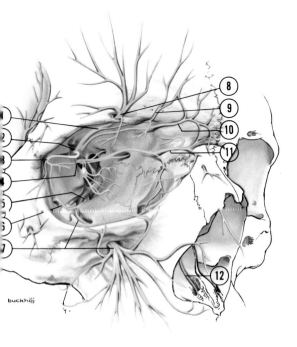

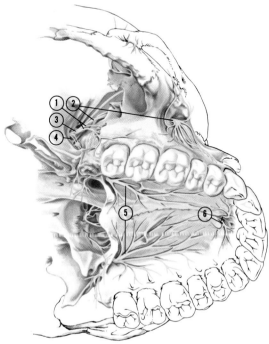

buckhöj

pect of the gum; 4) *the infraorbital nerve,* the direct continuation of the stem of the maxillary nerve, reaches the orbit through the inferior orbital fissure. It runs forward along the floor of the orbit giving off the *superior alveolar nerves* to the teeth and gum of the upper jaw (fig. 27, 49), af-

ter which it emerges through the infraorbital foramen to divide into branches to supply the skin between the palpebral fissure and the nostril (fig. 50, 51).

THE MANDIBULAR NERVE

The mandibular nerve is a mixed, although mainly sensory, nerve (fig. 49, 52). It leaves the cranial cavity through the foramen ovale and runs down in the infratemporal fossa. Here is gives off first its motor branches which supply all the muscles of mastication and the sensory *buccal nerve* which runs down on the outside of the buccinator muscle, which it perforates with numerous branches to supply the gum between the second molar and the second premolar teeth. After this, *the mandibular nerve* divides up into the following sensory nerves: 1) *the auriculotemporal nerve* which first lies medial to the neck of the mandible, but then at the posterior edge of the latter it turns sharply upwards immediately anterior to the external auditory canal and innervates the skin of the temple as well as that of the external auditory canal and of part of the auditory concha; 2) *the lingual nerve* runs down, lying between the ramus of the mandible and the medial pterygoid muscle. It curves forward at the anterior edge of this muscle to form an arc whose convex aspect points downwards and backwards where it enters the tongue from below to innervate its anterior two-thirds; 3) *the inferior alveolar nerve* which commences by bending downwards immediately behind *the lingual nerve,* but soon enters the mandibular foramen and transverses the mandibular canal while giving off branches to the teeth and gums of the lower jaw. A side-branch, *the mental nerve,* emerges through the mental foramen and innervates the skin of the underlip and lower jaw. The skin distribution is illustrated in fig. 54.

Fig. 52

1. Trigeminal n.
2. Gasserian ganglion
3. Mandibular n.
4. Buccal n.
5. Maxillary n.
6. Ophthalmic n.
7. Auriculotemporal n.
8. Inferior alveolar n.
9. Lingual n.
10. Mental n.

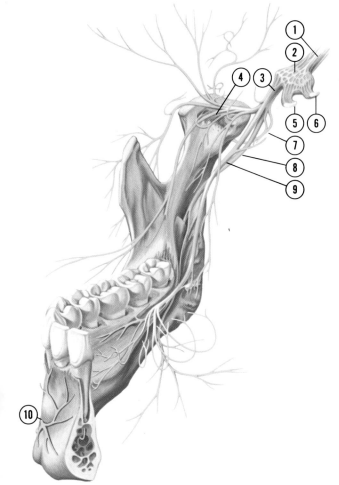

Block of the Gasserian Ganglion

Bertil Löfström

ANATOMY

The Gasserian ganglion which is situated intracranially, is located in the medial part of the middle cranial fossa. It lies lateral to the internal carotid artery and the cavernous sinus and slightly posterior and superior to the foramen ovale, through which the *mandibular nerve* leaves the cranium. With the technique described here, a needle is inserted upwards through the foramen ovale and into the cavum Meckelii which is formed by a separation of the two layers of the dura enclosing the ganglion.

The foramen ovale, a 5 mm. long canal with a maximum diameter of about 8 mm. is situated dorsally on the infratemporal and level surface of the greater wing of the sphenoid bone, immediately dorsolateral to the base of the pterygoid process (fig. 53).

TECHNIQUE

The patient is placed in the supine position, with the head raised by a pillow. He is requested to look straight ahead and to fix his gaze on a point marked on the wall. The mid-point of the zygomatic arch and the position of the articular tubercle are marked on the skin (fig. 55). A skin-weal is raised approximately 3 cm. lateral to the corner of the mouth, and on a level with the second

Fig. 53

Fig. 54

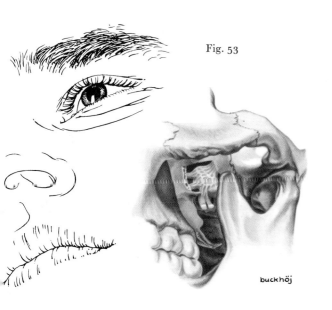

buckhöj

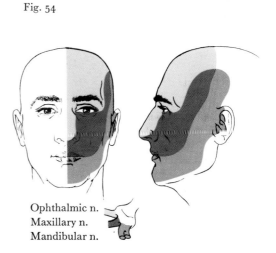

Ophthalmic n.
Maxillary n.
Mandibular n.

upper molar. The anaesthetist has to endeavour to insert the needle through the skin-weal in the direction of the pupil fixed as described, so as to make contact with bone immediately anterior to the foramen ovale. The needle is then directed more dorsally until paraesthesia is elicited and/or the needle slips into the foramen ovale.

A fine needle, 7-8 cm. long (possibly a fine spinal needle with stilette) with a rubber marker should be used. The needle is inserted first in the direction of the fixed pupil and towards the point marked on the mid-point of the zygomatic arch when viewed from the side. Contact with bone is usually obtained at a depth of 5 cm. from the skin, so the marker should be positioned on the needle at a distance of 5 cm. from its point. The point of the needle passes immediately lateral to the maxilla and the pterygoid process. Contact is made with bone on the infratemporal surface of the greater wing of the sphenoid, immediately anterior to the foramen ovale (fig. 56). When bone-contact has been made, the marker is moved

back 1.5 cm. from the skin. Then the needle is drawn out and reinserted in a more dorsal direction, towards the surface marking of the articular tubercle on the zygomatic process (but still directed towards the pupil, when viewed anteriorly). It may be necessary to adjust the position of the needle slightly, before paraesthesia is elicited and the foramen ovale reached. Paraesthesia should radiate towards the lower jaw. The needle is inserted a further 0.5 cm. – i.e. until the marker touches the skin and thus the point of the needle comes to lie in Meckel's cave, in or immediately adjacent to the Gasserian ganglion. Should paraesthesia be pronounced, 1 ml. of 2 % lignocaine may be injected before the needle is inserted further. When the needle has been correctly positioned (fig. 57) and following aspiration 2 ml. of 2 % lignocaine are injected. Complete block of the trigeminal nerve is obtained within 5-10 minutes.

Absolute alcohol is not injected until 15 minutes have elapsed following the injection of lignocaine and the dose must not exceed

Fig. 55

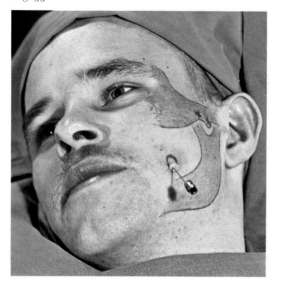

Fig. 56

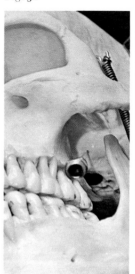

Fig. 57

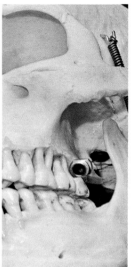

1 ml. A smaller dose of alcohol injected just inside the foramen ovale results in a more limited destruction of nerve tissue which usually does not involve the ophthalmic nerve, but is limited to the area illustrated in fig. 54.

INDICATIONS

This technique may be used with advantage for blocking the third branch of the trigeminal nerve or the Gasserian ganglion itself prior to unilateral surgery of the mandible or the face. A Gasserian ganglion block is of special value for facial surgery when general anaesthesia is considered undesirable, or when no other form of block is suitable.

Trigeminal Neuralgia: Basically, trigeminal neuralgia should be an indication for neurosurgery. However, if this cannot be performed within a reasonable time, or if the patient is greatly distressed by violent pain, a Gasserian ganglion block should be attempted. N.B. It is thought that the injection of absolute alcohol into the Gasserian ganglion may complicate subsequent neurosurgery.

COMPLICATIONS

Haematoma in the cheek is not unusual.

Subarachnoid injection, blocking the nerves at the base of the skull and the upper cervical roots. This in turn results in rapid unconsciousness. Respiratory paralysis and cardiovascular collapse may also occur. The prognosis is very favourable if the patient is immediately placed in the Trendelenburg position, artificial ventilation with oxygen instituted and a vasoconstrictor substance such as ephedrine, methoxamine or noradrenaline is administered as an intravenous drip. A subarachnoid injection may occur in spite of a negative aspiration test. Absolute alcohol must not be administered before a test dose of 2 % local anaesthetic solution has been shown to produce the desired result, without complications.

Keratitis readily occurs if the eye is not protected following anaesthesia of the ophthalmic nerve. If absolute alcohol has been injected, corneal sensitivity should be checked after the effect of the local anaesthetic has worn off.

Block of Branches of the Ophthalmic Nerve

ÅKE WÅHLIN

The Supraorbital and Supratrochlear Nerves

ANATOMY

The supraorbital nerve, which comes from the frontal nerve (fig. 49 and 50) divides in the orbit into medial and lateral branches, which emerge through two holes or notches beside the upper border of the orbit approximately 2.5 cm. from the mid-line, after which they are distributed to the forehead and up to the scalp (fig. 54, 58).

The supratrochlear nerve is also a branch of *the frontal nerve* (fig. 49, 50). The nerve runs forward by the upper medial corner of the aditus orbitae (fig. 58) and supplies mainly the skin of the medial part of the forehead.

TECHNIQUE

The supraorbital nerve. The site of the exit of the nerve at the upper border of the orbit is palpated. Using a fine, short needle, the nerve is sought for (fig. 58, 59) until para-

Fig. 58

1. Lateral branch of the frontal n.
2. Medial branch of the frontal n.
3. Supratrochlear n.

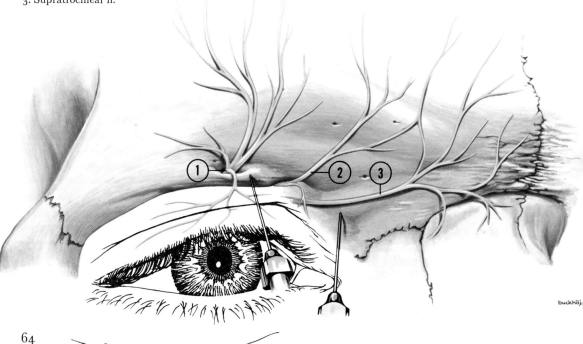

64

esthesia is obtained. This will be experienced by the patient mostly in the lateral part of the forehead. Then 1-3 ml. of prilocaine 1-2 % or lignocaine 1-2 % with vasoconstrictor are injected.

The supratrochlear nerve. A short fine needle is inserted immediately below the angle between the superior and medial borders of the

Fig. 59

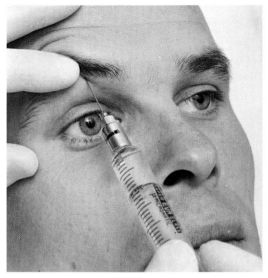

Fig. 60

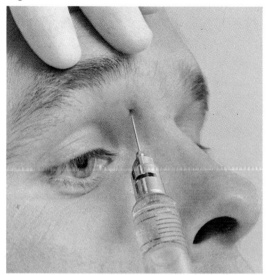

orbit, where the nerve is found at the medial edge of the root of the nose (fig. 58, 60). The nerve is sought until paraesthesia is obtained over the central part of the forehead, and 1-3 ml. prilocaine 1-2 % or lignocaine 1-2% with vasoconstrictor are injected.

The branches of the supratrochlear and supraorbital nerves may be blocked more easily by raising a weal over the root of the nose, after which the point of the needle is advanced under the skin immediately above and along the entire eyebrow (fig. 61) while 3-6 ml. of prilocaine 1-2 % or lignocaine 1-2 % with vasoconstrictor are being injected. Anaesthesia of the other side may be produced from the same skin-weal.

INDICATIONS

For surgical interventions on the forehead the latter method is preferred because of its simplicity. However, the selective method is more suitable for differential diagnosis of trigger zones in the area of distribution of the trigeminal nerve, since from the area of distribution, the paraesthesia elicited confirms that the respective nerve has been found.

Both methods are equally suitable for block in cases of post-traumatic pain.

Fig. 61

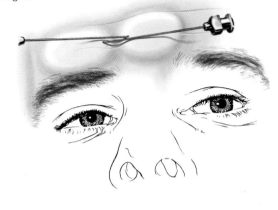

Block of Branches of the Maxillary Nerve

Åke Wåhlin

The Infraorbital Nerve

ANATOMY

The *infraorbital nerve* constitutes the direct continuation of the *maxillary nerve*. It enters the orbit through the inferior orbital fissure and runs forward lying first in the sulcus and then within the infraorbital canal, finally emerging through the infraorbital foramen. Here it divides to supply the skin of the lower eye-lid, the side of the nose and the upper lip, along with the mucous membrane lining the nasal vestibule. (Fig. 49, 50, 51, 62).

INTRAORAL ROUTE

The midpoint of the lower border of the orbit is first palpated by the middle finger of one hand, which is then moved carefully to a point approximately one centimetre lower down (fig. 63). In most patients the neurovascular bundle issuing from the infraorbital foramen may be palpated here. The middle finger remains over the infraorbital foramen and using the thumb and index

Fig. 62

1. Infraorbital n.
2. Palpebral branches

Fig. 63

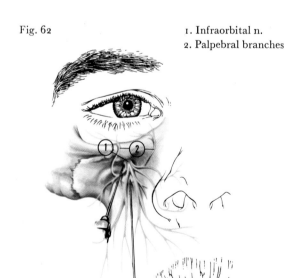

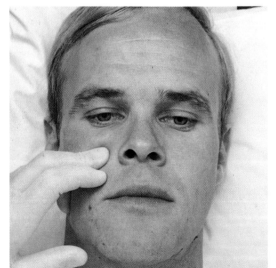

finger, the upper lip is elevated. A needle with syringe attached is inserted by the other hand into the mucous membrane at its reflection from the upper gum, until its point comes to lie under the tip of the middle finger (fig. 64). Should the point of the needle be impalpable, the swelling of the tissues as local anaesthetic solution is injected can be felt by the finger-tip. Here 2-3 ml. of lignocaine or prilocaine 2 % are injected.

EXTRAORAL ROUTE

The needle is inserted into the skin approximately 1 cm. below the point palpated when the intraoral technique is being used, and directed slowly towards the infraorbital foramen (fig. 65). Paraesthesia in the area of distribution of the nerve is not unfrequently elicited, a fact of which the patient should be informed. Aspiration is attempted, to avoid injection into the neighbouring artery and vein and the same quantity of solution is injected as with the intraoral technique.

The needle should not be inserted into the canal, unless this is clearly indicated, since injection into the canal can result in lesions of the nerves with prolonged discomfort.

INDICATIONS

Surgical interference in the area supplied by the infraorbital nerve.

Differential diagnosis in neuralgia of the trigger zones in this part of the trigeminal nerve.

Complicated extraction with flap resection of one or more of the incisors or the canine as well as of operative treatment of a root-cyst or granuloma.

Fig. 64

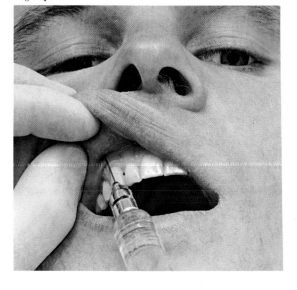

Fig. 65

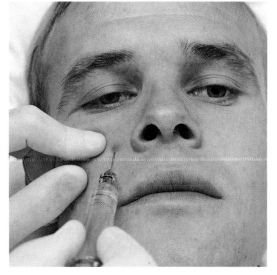

The Superior Alveolar Branches, the Great Palatine and the Nasopalatine Nerves

ANATOMY

The superior alveolar branches arise from *the infraorbital nerve.* Before this nerve has even passed the inferior orbital fissure, it gives off *the posterior superior alveolar branches,* which run down on the maxillary tuberosity, where they enter to supply the molars of the upper jaw (fig. 51, 66). While the infraorbital nerve lies in the infraorbital canal, it gives off *the middle superior alveolar branch* and several *anterior superior alveolar branches* (fig. 49), which innervate the premolar, canine and incisor teeth.

The great palatine nerve (fig. 49, 51) runs from the pterygopalatine fossa down through the pterygopalatine canal and emerges through the greater palatine foramen into the hard palate to supply its mucous membrane, as well as the palatal aspect of the gingiva.

The nasopalatine nerve is the largest of the posterior superior nasal branches (fig. 49, 50, 51). It runs downwards and forwards along the nasal septum and gives off branches through the incisive canal to the anterior part of the hard palate and the adjacent gum margin of the upper incisors.

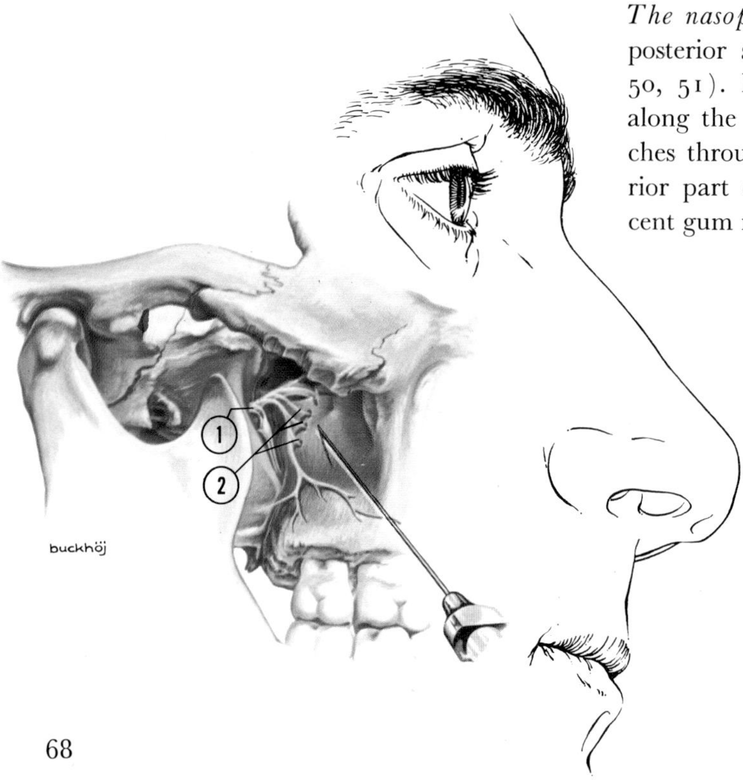

buckhöj

Fig. 66

1. Maxillary n.
2. Posterior superior alveolar branches

The posterior superior alveolar branches are blocked by an injection administered behind the infrazygomatic crest and immediately distal to the second molar tooth. After its insertion, the tip of the needle is advanced right up to the maxillary tuberosity, approximately 2-3 cm. in a flat arc with its concave side upwards, while approximately 2 ml. prilocaine 2 % or lignocaine 2 % with or without a vasoconstrictor are injected. This technique is known as a tuberosity injection (fig. 66).

The middle superior and anterior superior alveolar branches (fig. 27) are blocked in the following way. The needle is inserted into the buccal fold opposite the tooth to be anaesthetized, directing the tip of the needle towards the point where the apex of the root of the tooth is thought to lie (fig. 67). Here 1-2 ml. of prilocaine 2 % or lignocaine 2 % with or without adrenaline are injected, while the point of the needle is moved fan-wise, slightly and very carefully. In this way up to three teeth may be blocked from the same point of insertion.

The great palatine nerve is blocked with a few tenths of a ml. of prilocaine 2 % or lignocaine 2 %, with or without vasoconstrictor, in or immediately adjacent to the greater palatine foramen, which may be found at the level of the 2nd molar, 1 cm above the gingival margin (fig. 68).

The nasopalatine nerve is blocked with a few tenths of a ml. of prilocaine 2 % or lignocaie 2 %, with or without vasoconstrictor, in or immediately adjacent to the incisive canal, which reaches the middle line immediately behind the incisors (fig. 69).

INDICATIONS

The intraoral technique is usually employed in dentistry, to anaesthetize teeth in the upper jaw. For conservative treatment, which as a rule only requires analgesia of the pulp, an injection into the buccal fold is sufficient. For surgical interventions this must be supplemented by a palatal injection for the respective tooth. Extraction of all the teeth of one half of the jaw requires anaesthesia of both the great palatine and the nasopalatine nerves.

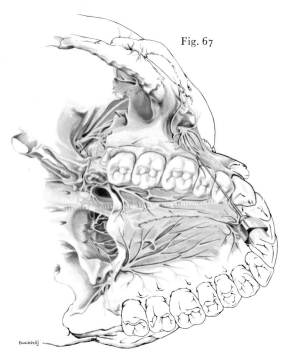

Fig. 67

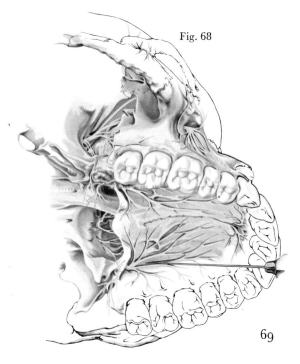

Fig. 68

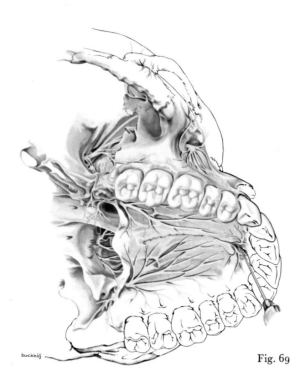

Fig. 69

The site of insertion is the point of intersection of the lower border of the zygoma and the anterior border of the mandibular ramus (fig. 70-I). The needle is directed slightly upwards and somewhat backwards and inserted as far as the maxillary tuberosity. Still in contact with the tuberosity, the needle is inserted further until the needle leaves the convexity of the tuberosity and stops when contact with the greater wing of the sphenoid has been made (fig. 70-II). Here approximately 4 ml. of 2 % prilocaine or 2 % lignocaine, with or without vasoconstrictor, are injected.

INDICATIONS

Surgical interventions involving the skin of the side of the nose, the lower eye-lid and the upper lip; the bone of the jaw with the maxillary sinus and the alveolar process, including the teeth and finally the mucoperiosteum of the palate and the buccal fold. For more extensive surgery of the maxilla general anaesthesia should be considered.

Fig. 70

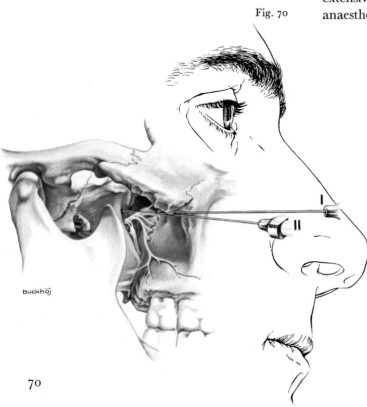

Block of Branches of the Mandibular Nerve

Åke Wåhlin

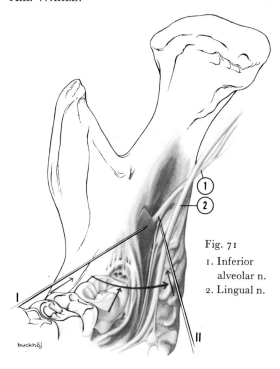

Fig. 71

1. Inferior alveolar n.
2. Lingual n.

Intraoral Block of the Inferior Alveolar Nerve

ANATOMY

The *mandibular nerve* divides immediately below the foramen ovale. From here, the *inferior alveolar nerve* runs downwards, lying first medially to the lateral pterygoid muscle. It then runs lateral to the medial pterygoid muscle, between it and the inner aspect of the ramus of the mandible. The nerve now proceeds through the mandibular foramen, which is situated at approximately the mid-point of the ramus. The nerve goes through the mandibular canal until it lies at the level of the medial incisor. Here it divides, giving off branches to supply the teeth and gums of the lower jaw (fig. 52, 71).

TECHNIQUE

The anterior border of the ramus of the mandible, the oblique line, is located with the left index finger. The needle is inserted at a point immediately medial to this, and approximately 1 cm. above the occlusal surface of the third molar. The syringe must lie virtually parallel to the body of the mandible and *parallel to the occlusal surfaces of the*

Fig. 72

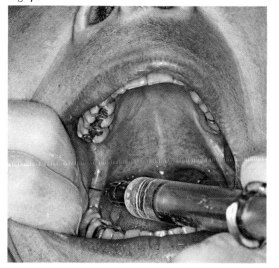

Fig. 73

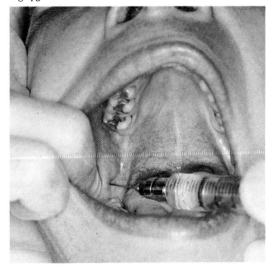

teeth of the lower jaw. From this original position (fig. 72) the needle is slowly advanced along the medial side of the ramus to a depth of 2 cm. (fig. 71 I), whilst the syringe is rotated simultaneously over to the premolar region of the opposite side of the mandible, all the time maintaining the same horizontal plane (fig. 73). The needle must remain in contact with the ramus while this manoeuvre is being performed.

A higher success rate will be achieved if the patient's mouth remains wide open all the time. If a block of the lingual nerve is required as well then a small quantity of solution is deposited as the needle passes the oblique line (fig. 71 II). In actual fact it is difficult to avoid blocking the lingual nerve, since a small quantity of solution should be injected while the needle is being advanced. When the needle is in the correct position, 1.5-2 ml. prilocaine or lignocaine 2 % with or without vasoconstrictor should be injected.

This nerve-block may also be performed by inserting the needle with the syringe in the final position described and advancing it directly to the ramus. This technique, however, needs greater experience.

In edentulous patients, it is especially important to locate the landmarks mentioned and to keep the syringe in the correct horizontal plain.

For extractions in the molar region the periosteum and mucous membrane on the buccal side of the molars must be anaesthetized. This may be performed by injecting 0.5-1.0 ml. of prilocaine or lignocaine 2 % with or without vasoconstrictor into the cheek, immediately above its junction with the gum, opposite the third molar (fig. 75), thus blocking the buccal nerve (fig. 52, 74).

INDICATIONS

The intraoral route is most suitable for oral surgery, and conservative dentistry in the

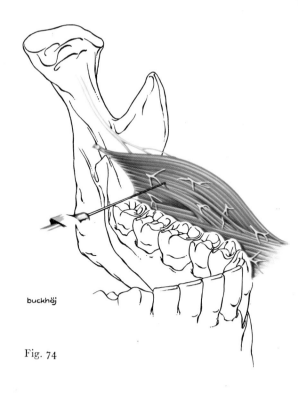

buckhöj

Fig. 74

Fig. 75

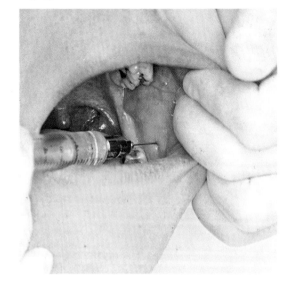

lower jaw. Note that the block can be incomplete in the incisor area, owing to its bilateral innervation.

Unilateral operative surgery on the lingual aspect of the alveolar process, in the sulcus from the first molar to almost the midline, and if the lingual nerve has been blocked as well, operations on the lateral border of the tongue. When supplemented by blocking the buccal nerve, operations in the region of the sulcus corresponding to the 2nd and 3rd molars, as well as extraction of these teeth. A bilateral block should not be performed in out-patient practice.

Extraoral Block of the Inferior Alveolar Nerve

ANATOMY

The mandibular branch of the *trigeminal nerve* leaves the foramen ovale and lies along the floor of the infratemporal fossa anterior to the medial meningeal artery (fig. 76) and is covered by the masseter and lateral pterygoid muscles.

TECHNIQUE

The needle is inserted into the space formed by the zygomatic arch and the incisura mandibulae and immediately anterior to the head of the mandible, with the mouth open to its widest extent (fig. 76). The needle is advanced at right angles to the skin as far as the base of the infratemporal fossa. The nerve is encountered at a depth of 2-3 cm., lying 1.0-1.5 cm., in front of the foramen ovale where 3-4 ml. of prilocaine or lignocaine 1-2 % with vasoconstrictor are injected.

INDICATIONS

Dental and surgical operations on the lower jaw, as well as its mucous membrane and periosteum on both its buccal and lingual aspects and the anterior two-thirds of the tongue with the lower part of the cheek. However, general anaesthesia is to be preferred when more extensive surgery is to be performed.

This form of anaesthesia is suitable for such patients who, because of pain or swell-

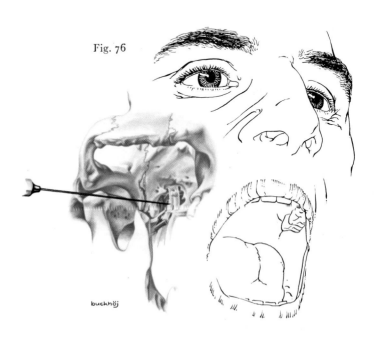

Fig. 76

buckhöj

73

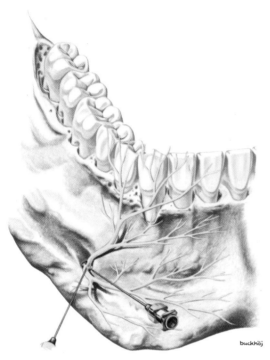

Fig. 77

ing, cannot open their mouths sufficiently for the performance of an intraoral block.

The Mental Nerve

ANATOMY

The *mental nerve* arises in the mandibular canal from the *inferior alveolar nerve,* and issues from the mental foramen on a level with the second premolar (fig. 77). The nerve supplies the skin and mucous membrane of the lower lip, together with the skin of the jaw.

INTRAORAL ROUTE

The mental foramen is situated inside the lower lip at its junction with the lower gum, just posterior to the 1st premolar tooth. The left index finger is used to palpate the point where the neurovascular bundle issues from the mandible and to maintain light pressure on it. Meanwhile the needle is inserted from the side until its point is felt in close relation to the neuromuscular bundle (fig. 78) where 1-2 ml. prilocaine or lignocaine 2 % with or without vasoconstrictor are injected. Vascular injury is avoided by this technique.

Fig. 78

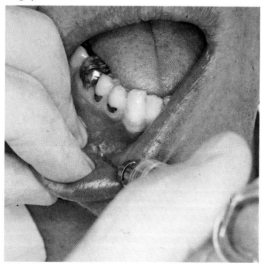

Fig. 79

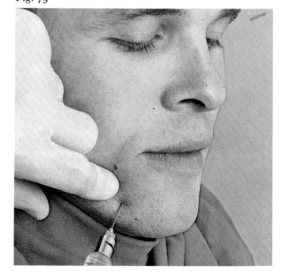

The insertion of the needle into the mental foramen to obtain better anaesthesia is not to be recommended because of the risk of inducing nerve-injury and subsequent numbness of the lower lip. Should it not be possible to position the needle exactly, adequate anaesthesia can often be obtained by depositing solution around the mental foramen.

EXTRAORAL ROUTE

The neurovascular bundle issuing from the mental foramen can usually be palpated from outside. Thus much the same technique is used as for intraoral injection (fig. 79).

The anaesthetized area stretches to the midline of the mandible, both when the extraoral or the intraoral technique is used. Both techniques may be used unilaterally or bilaterally, depending on the extent of the proposed operation.

The nerves to a single incisor may also be blocked by submucous infiltration in the sulcus opposite to the tooth to be treated (fig. 80, 81).

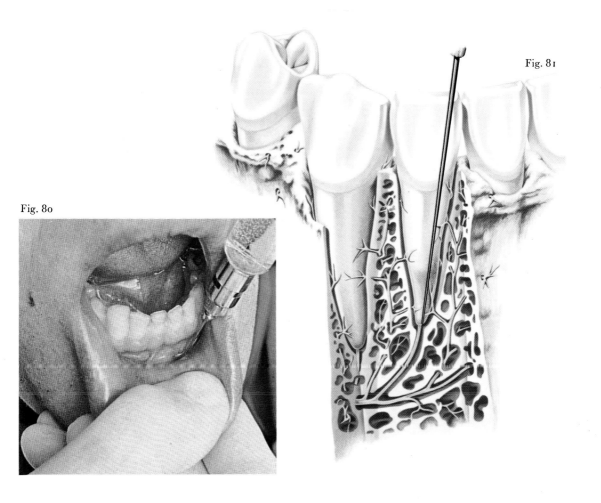

Fig. 81

Fig. 80

75

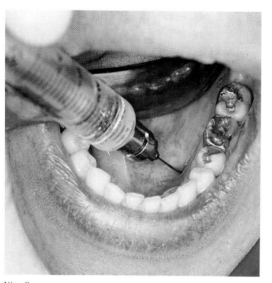

Fig. 82

However, extractions can only be carried out following supplementary anaesthesia of the lingual nerve. This is achieved by injecting a small amount of local anaesthetic on the lingual aspect, immediately behind the tooth to be extracted (fig. 82, 83).

INDICATIONS

Treatment of the incisor, canine or first premolar teeth of the lower jaw. Surgery of the lower lip, the mucous membrane as it is reflected from the gum, or the labial part of the alveolar process.

Extractions in the above mentioned group of teeth can be performed after supplementary anaesthesia of the lingual nerve.

Fig. 83

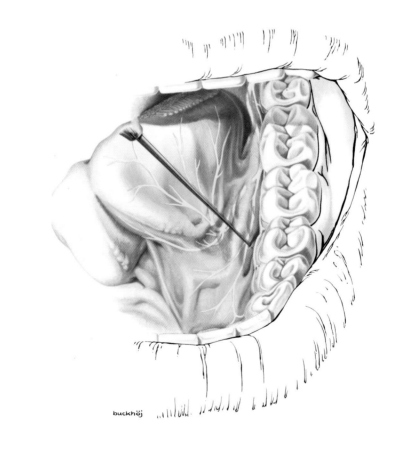

buckhöj

Cervical Nerve Block

Bertil Löfström

ANATOMY

On leaving the respective intervertebral foramina *the cervical nerves* pass behind the vertebral artery and lie with their anterior branches in the nerve sulci of the transverse processes (fig. 84). These can usually be palpated immediately posterior to the sternocleidomastoid muscle. The anterior branches of the first four cervical nerves join together just lateral to the transverse processes, to form the *cervical plexus*.

Fig. 84

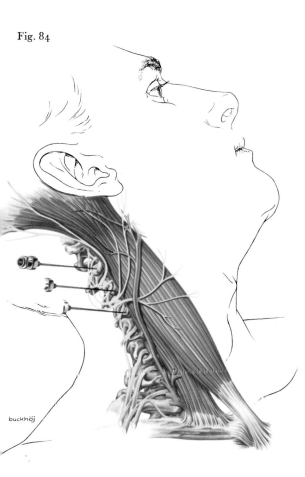

buckhöj

TECHNIQUE

The anterior branches of the cervical nerves are blocked in the sulci of the transverse processes. The patient is placed in the supine position with the head turned away from the side to be blocked. At the same time, the head is bent somewhat backwards.

The mastoid process, the most caudal point of which lies just cranial to the first cervical vertebra, is marked, together with the transverse process of the sixth cervical vertebra. This is the easiest transverse process to palpate and is found usually on the same level as the thyroid cartilage. A straight line is drawn between these two points. The transverse process of the second cervical vertebra can usually be palpated 1.5 cm. caudal to the mastoid process, and 0.75 cm. dorsal to the line already drawn. Then the transverse processes of C3, C4 and C5 are sought and palpated; they lie about 1.5 cm. from each other. The transverse processes of all the above vertebræ should be marked before the block is begun (fig. 85).

The anaesthetist will find it most convenient to stand beside the patient's head. A fine-gauge needle, 5 cm. long, is inserted, guided by a palpating finger, towards the transverse process. The distance between the skin and each transverse process is from 1.5-3 cm. The needle is inserted perpendicular to the skin, and pointing somewhat caudally, so as to avoid the risk of the needle slipping upwards along the transverse process and into the intervertebral foramen, where the dura could be perforated and a subarachnoid injection of local anaesthetic be given. The point of the needle must be placed in or adjacent to the nerve sulcus if good anaesthesia is to be obtained. If the anaesthetist is not certain that the needle is so positioned, he should move its point on the transverse process until paraesthesia is obtained. Should such be obtained, 3 ml. lignocaine 0.5-1 %

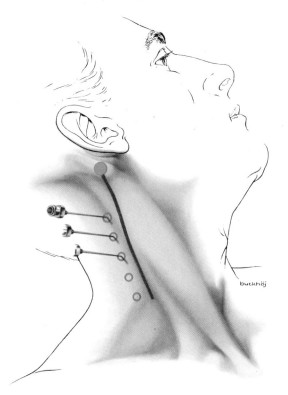

Fig. 85

with vasoconstrictor is injected against each nerve. In the absence of paraesthesia, 7 ml. of 0.5-1.0 % solution are injected with the point of the needle in contact with the transverse process and 3 ml. as the needle is withdrawn. The area innervated by the cervical nerves 2-5 is illustrated in fig. 86. For surgical anaesthesia it is an advantage to block the superficial cervical plexus as well. For this purpose a needle is inserted at the level of C3 and local anaesthetic solution is injected along the posterior margin of the sternocleidomastoid muscle.

INDICATIONS

Operations on the thyroid. Investigations of pain – in the case, for example, of cervical spondylosis. In such cases the point of the needle can be moved in cranially towards the intervertebral foramen. When paraesthesia

has been induced, 2-4 ml. of a 2 % solution of lignocaine with vasoconstrictor are injected in order to make sure that anaesthesia reaches as far as or even beyond the nerve section which is under pressure.

N.B. Risk of penetrating the dural cuff around the nerve root.

COMPLICATIONS

Since the neck is a very vascular region, *intravascular injection* can easily occur. It should be realized that the needle can reach the vertebral artery (cf. stellate ganglion block, p. 141). *Cervical sympathetic block* resulting in a Horner syndrome is not uncommon. *Paralysis of the phrenic nerve* will occur frequently on the anaesthetized side, with subsequent cessation of diaphragmatic movement. *Hoarseness,* caused by diffusion of the local anaesthetic to the recurrent laryngeal nerve can occur. *Subarachnoid injection* with resulting high spinal anaesthesia. (Tilt the patient head down, ventilate him with oxygen and, if necessary, give a vasopressor intravenously).

Fig. 86

C 2
C 3
C 4
C 5

Brachial Plexus Block - Supraclavicular Approach

Ejnar Eriksson

ANATOMY

The *Brachial Plexus* is formed by the fusion of the anterior rami of C5, C6, C7, C8 and T1, in addition to a smaller contribution from C4 and T2 (fig. 87). The plexus stretches from the lateral aspect of the cervical vertebral column downwards and laterally, running together with the subclavian artery between the scalenus anterior and scalenus medius muscles. It then passes behind the mid-point of the clavicle above the first rib to reach the axillary fossa. Here the brachial plexus joins up to form three main cords which are situated medially, laterally and dorsally to the axillary artery. Topographically, a supraclavicular and an infraclavicular part of the brachial plexus may be distinguished.

TECHNIQUE

Supraclavicular brachial plexus block is performed where the plexus crosses the first rib.

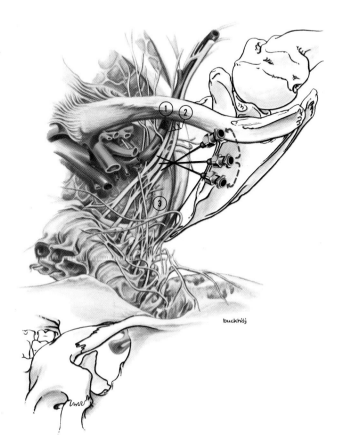

Fig. 87
1. Subclavian a.
2. Brachial plexus
3. First rib

79

Here the three divisions of the plexus are relatively easily located. The patient lies with his head turned towards the opposite side. A skin weal is raised 1 cm. over and immediately lateral to the midpoint of the clavicle. (fig. 88). A 5 cm long *fine*-gauge needle is inserted at an angle of about 80° to the skin (fig. 89). Cautiously the needle is directed somewhat caudally until contact is made either with one of the divisions of the brachial plexus (when the patient feels paraesthesia extending into the arm) or with the first rib. Since the risk of puncturing the pleura is always present with this approach contact should be sought with the first rib. When this has been found, the needle is carefully moved along the rib until paraesthesia is elicited (fig. 91). It is best to explore for all three main divisions of the plexus, thus eliciting paraesthesia in the upper arm, lower arm, and both sides of the hand. Approximately 8-10 ml. of a 1.5 %

solution of lignocaine or prilocaine with vasoconstrictor are injected into each division. Coughing by the patient while paraesthesia is being sought may indicate pleural puncture, and the procedure must be discontinued. A chest X-ray will reveal any possible pneumathorax. However, since a pneumothorax may develop slowly, the patient should be admitted to hospital and observed for 24 hours, even if the initial X-ray is normal. (The axillary approach to the brachial plexus eliminates the risk of pleural puncture cf. p. 82). The danger of intravascular injection is also present; therefore careful aspiration tests are essential. Puncture of the subclavian artery indicates that the needle has been inserted too far medially. The plexus should be sought more laterally. The area of sensory anaesthesia following supraclavicular brachial plexus block is demonstrated in fig. 90.

Fig. 88

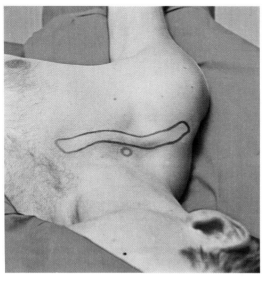

Fig. 89

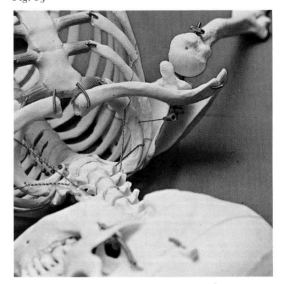

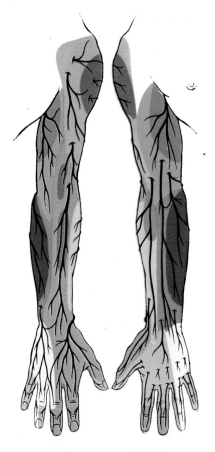

DOSAGE

25-30 ml. lignocaine or prilocaine 1 %-1.5 %, with vasoconstrictor. Good anaesthesia can also be obtained by using 40-50 ml. of 0.5 % lignocaine or prilocaine with vaso-constrictor. If this concentration is used at least 15 ml. are injected at the site of each of the three main divisions of the plexus.

CONTRAINDICATIONS

Relative contraindications are children, in whom the axillary approach should be used instead; tall, narrow-chested patients, who often have the apex of their pleurae situated at a high level. Bilateral supraclavicular brachial plexus block should not be performed, because of the risk of bilateral pneumothorax.

Fig. 90

Upper lateral cutaneous n. of the arm (axillary n.)

Medial cutaneous n. of the arm

Radial n.

Lateral cutaneous n. of the forearm (musculocutaneous n.)

Medial cutaneous n. of the forearm

Median n.

Ulnar n.

Fig. 91

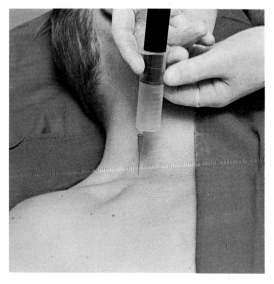

Brachial Plexus Block - Axillary Approach

Ejnar Eriksson

ANATOMY

The *brachial plexus* (from C5, C6, C7, C8, T1 and some fibres from C4 and T2) passes between the clavicle and the first rib, and extends in this way from the neck to the axilla. The infraclavicular section surrounds the axillary artery with three bundles, a medial, lateral and posterior, from which the long nerves of the upper limb arise. The axillary artery is accompanied, on its medial side, by the axillary vein. In the axillary fossa these vessels and the brachial plexus are enveloped in a common, fairly taut sheath of connective tissue (fig. 92). Since all the long branches of the brachial plexus lie collected in a relatively narrow fascial tube between the axilla and the proximal part of the upper arm, an axillary approach is possible.

However, it should be noted that *the musculocutaneous nerve*, carrying sensory fibres to the radial side of the forearm, leaves the brachial plexus high up in the axillary fossa. Therefore, this is the most difficult branch to block by this method (fig. 92, arrow).

TECHNIQUE

With the patient lying with the arm abducted at an angle of about 90° the axillary artery is palpated and a *short* (4-5 cm.) needle is inserted towards and slightly above it (fig. 93). Here the plexus lies superficially; failure to appreciate this fact and consequent deep injection is the most common cause of failure. Arterial puncture should be avoided since a haematoma in the fascial sheath reduces the success rate of this technique.

If the needle shows marked pulsation, it indicates that its point lies near the artery in the correct fascial compartment. After careful aspiration the anaesthetic solution is then injected bearing in mind the patient's body weight and general condition. Paraesthesia is not sought using this technique. However,

Fig. 92

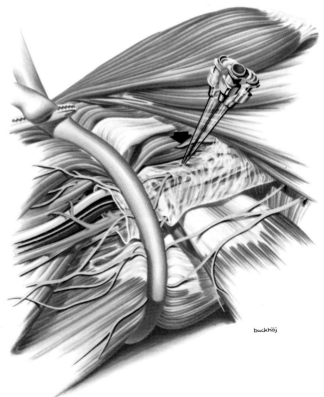

buckhöj

should it be encountered the needle point is in the correct position, but injection must not be attempted until the point has been withdrawn slightly. In very obese patients it is an advantage to elicite paraesthesiae. All local anaesthetic agents are lipoid soluble and in such patients an unusual quantity may be absorbed by the fatty tissue instead of difusing to the nerve.

A tourniquet applied to the upper arm just below the axilla prevents the anaesthetic solution from spreading distally (fig. 94) and forces it upwards (Eriksson, 1965). Thus the chance of producing a successful block of the musculocutaneous nerve is considerably increased (fig. 95) and at the same time the volume of local anaesthetic injected may be reduced. The tourniquet should remain in place for about ten minutes.

Induction time is longer with an axillary than with a supraclavicular plexus block, because the local anaesthetic must diffuse to all the branches of the brachial plexus. This may take up to 25-30 minutes in an adult, in children somewhat less. The advantage of

this technique is that there is no risk of pneumothorax, which makes this method most suitable for outpatient use. The area of anaesthesia following an axillary brachial plexus block is demonstrated in fig. 96. The duration of the anaesthesia can easily be prolonged if an epidural catheter is introduced into the fascial sheath and repeated doses are given through it.

Fig. 94

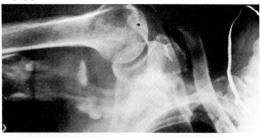

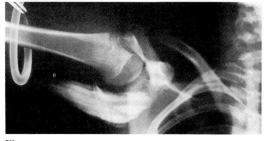

Fig. 95
Fig. 96

Fig. 93

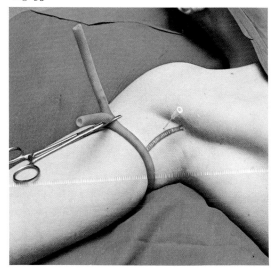

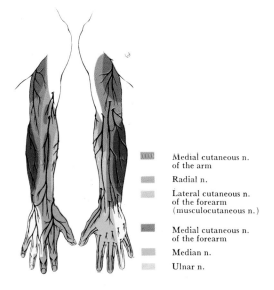

    Medial cutaneous n. of the arm

    Radial n.

    Lateral cutaneous n. of the forearm (musculocutaneous n.)

    Medial cutaneous n. of the forearm

    Median n.

    Ulnar n.

Well-developed (>80 kg.) males 25-30 ml. lignocaine or prilocaine 1.5 % with adrenaline 1:200,000.

Smaller males and females (50-70 kg.) 20-25 ml. lignocaine or prilocaine 1.5 % with adrenaline 1:200,000.

Teenagers (40-60 kg.) 15-20 ml. 1.5 % lignocaine or prilocaine with adrenaline 1:200,000.

Children, age group 8-12 years (25-35 kg.) 14-20 ml. 1.0 % lignocaine or prilocaine with adrenaline 1.200,000.

Children, age group 4-7 years (19-25 kg.) 9-14 ml. 1.0 % prilocaine with adrenaline 1:200,000.

Children, age group 1-3 years (8-18 kg.) 6-9 ml. 0.5-1.0 % prilocaine without adrenaline 1:200,000.

INDICATIONS

Operations on the hand, forearm and the distal part of the upper arm, especially in outpatients and industrial accidents. Axillary block produces excellent anaesthesia for the reduction of fractures in small children. These have often eaten just before they attend hospital and general anaesthesia would usually have to be preceded by emptying the stomach contents. A simple needle prick in the axilla is not infrequently less psychologically traumatic than general anaesthesia.

CONTRAINDICATIONS

Damage to or disease of the plexus or the distal nerves in the arm.

COMPLICATIONS

Arterial puncture, venipuncture. Careful aspiration and rotation of the needle prior to injection is therefore essential.

Suprascapular Nerve Block

Torsten Gordh

ANATOMY

The suprascapular nerve (C4, C5, C6) passes through the scapular notch to the supraspinous fossa, where it innervates the supraspinatus muscle. One branch continues past the neck of the scapula to supply the infraspinatus muscle. The nerve also gives off sensory fibres to the shoulder joint and surrounding structures (fig. 97).

TECHNIQUE

The patient is placed in the sitting position with the arms resting against the rail of a chair. The landmarks which are made use of are illustrated in fig. 98.

A line is drawn along the spine of the scapula and another line which divides the angle of the scapula into two. The scapular notch is situated on this second line, and approximately 1-2 cm. cranial to its point of intersection with the first line.

A weal is raised here. Using a 5 cm. long fine-gauge needle, contact is made with the supraspinatus fossa and the point of the needle is "walked" along this until the scapular notch is located. Following careful aspiration 2-3 ml. of lignocaine 1 % with adrenaline are injected here. This injection is performed at a depth of approximately 1.5 cm.

INDICATIONS

Diagnosis and treatment of painful conditions of the shoulder and the shoulder joint.

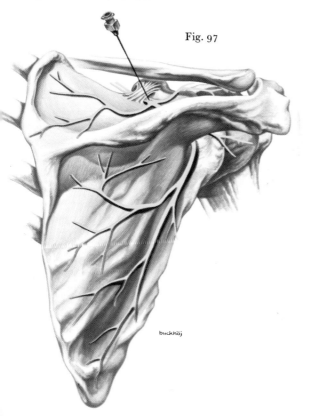

Fig. 97

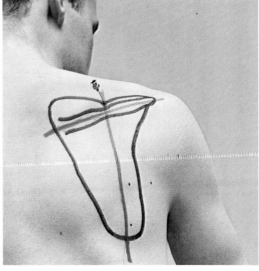

Fig. 98

Nerve Block at
the Elbow

BERTIL LÖFSTRÖM

The Ulnar Nerve

ANATOMY

The ulnar nerve (C6, C7, C8, T1) which in its course through the distal third of the upper arm has already perforated the medial intermuscular septum and entered the extensor compartment, passing the elbow in the ulnar nerve sulcus which is situated on the posterior aspect of the medial epicondyle of the humerus. Here it can usually be palpated without difficulty (fig. 99). After this, the nerve passes between the two heads of flexor carpi ulnaris muscle and continues downwards on the flexor aspect of the forearm. Occasionally the nerve is not found in its groove, but may be palpated further out on the medial epicondyle.

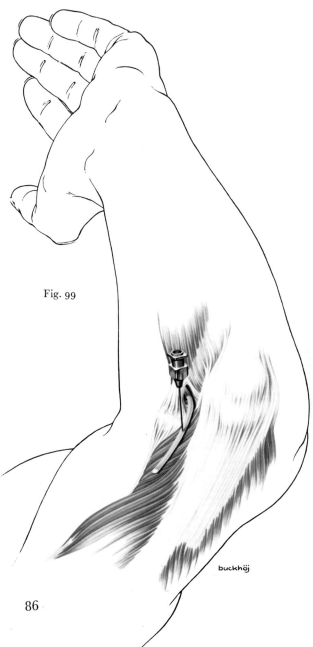

Fig. 99

buckhöj

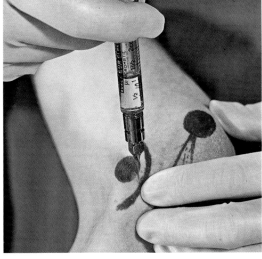

Fig. 100

TECHNIQUE

The nerve is most easily blocked where it runs in its groove behind the medial epicondyle of the humerus. Where possible, it is best to block the nerve 1-2 cm. proximal to the ulnar nerve sulcus, in order to avoid the risk of neuritis.

The nerve is palpated while the elbow is flexed to 90°. A very fine needle, (outer diameter 0.40-0.45 mm.) mounted on a 2-5 ml. syringe is inserted towards the nerve (fig. 100). When paraesthesia radiating down the ulnar side of the forearm and out into the little finger is elicited, the needle is fixed and 1-2 ml. of lignocaine 1 % with or without adrenaline are injected slowly i.e. over a period of 10-20 seconds. The nerve can also be blocked if the needle be positioned just outside the nerve, as determined by touch. In this case 5-10 ml. lignocaine 1 % with or without adrenaline are required for nerve block. This latter technique does not give the same reliable results as intraneural injection.

The cutaneous distribution of the ulnar nerve is illustrated in fig. 101.

Latency is short (less than 5 minutes) when the injection is an intraneural one but longer (15-30 minutes) for the extraneural technique.

INDICATIONS

Ulnar nerve block is useful when minor surgery is to be performed within the area of the nerve's distribution and for supplementing an inadequate supraclavicular block of the brachial plexus. Fibres from C8 and T1 are usually those most difficult to reach with this approach. Bilateral ulnar nerve block has been found very useful for testing local anaesthetic drugs (Albert & Löfström 1961, 1965 a, b).

CONTRAINDICATIONS

Ulnar nerve block should not be used in cases of ulnar nerve neuritis, nor when the characteristic significant paraesthesia can be elicited easily by palpating the nerve.

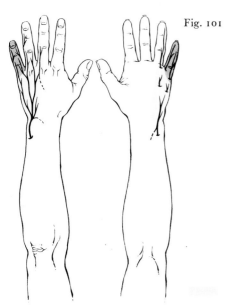

Fig. 101

Ulnar nerve

The Median Nerve

ANATOMY

The median nerve (C5, C6, C7, C8, T1) runs distally along the inner border of the upper arm, where it is included in the large neurovascular sheath. In the cubital fossa the nerve lies medial to the brachial artery and, covered by the aponeurosis of the biceps muscle, it runs between the two heads of pronator teres, continuing into the flexor compartment of the lower arm (fig. 102).

TECHNIQUE

The median nerve can best be blocked on the ulnar side of the brachial artery and on the same level as a line drawn between the two epicondyles. Here the nerve lies quite superficial and can be palpated in thin individuals. A short fine needle (S.W.G. 26-27) is inserted 0.5-0.75 cm. medial to the brachial artery. Often in order to elicite paraesthesia, the needle has to be moved fanwise up and down in a plane through the epicondyles and at right angles to the long axis of the arm (fig. 104).

When paraesthesia has been obtained, approximately 5 ml. of lignocaine 0.5-1.0 %, with or without adrenaline, is then injected. A subcutaneous infiltration is required to block the cutaneous branches in the forearm.

INDICATIONS

The area innervated by the median nerve is shown in fig. 103 and indicates the usefulness of this block for minor surgery.

Median nerve block may be used for full-thickness skin grafting on the three radial fingers of the hand. If subcutaneous infiltration right across the proximal part of the lower arm is also done, it is possible to use the palmar aspect as a donor area.

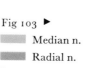

◄ Fig. 102
1. Median n.
2. Lateral cutaneous n.
   of the forearm
3. Radial n.
4. Brachial a.
5. Tendon of the biceps m.
6. Brachioradialis m.

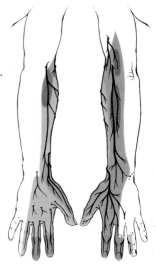

Fig 103 ►

　　Median n.

　　Radial n.

　　Lateral cutaneous
　　n. of the forearm

buckhöj

This block is usually contraindicated in cases of carpal tunnel syndrome and other forms of median nerve neuritis.

The Radial Nerve and the Lateral Cutaneous Nerve of the Forearm

ANATOMY

These nerves together supply the radial aspects of both the forearm and the back of the hand (fig. 103).

The *radial nerve* (C5, C6, C7, C8, T1) runs in the spiral groove around the posterio-lateral aspect of the humerus. It continues in front of the elbow-joint and comes to lie in the groove between the brachio-radialis and the biceps muscles (fig. 102). At the level of the head of the radius the nerve divides into a *deep ramus,* which is the motor supply of the whole of the extensor muscles of the forearm and a *superficial ramus,* which is sensory and follows the radial artery, eventually supplying the radial side of the back of the hand.

The *lateral cutaneous nerve of the forearm* (C5, C6, C7) which is the sensory continuation of the *musculocutaneous nerve,* perfora-

Fig. 104

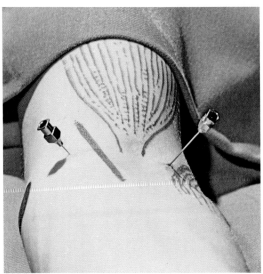

tes the deep fascia on the lateral side of the biceps muscle just proximal to the elbow-joint (fig. 102) and is distributed to the skin on the lateral side of the lower arm, as far down as the radiocarpal joint (fig. 103).

TECHNIQUE

The following technique may be used to block both nerves. At the level of the extended elbow-joint a fairly long fine-gauge needle is inserted between the brachioradialis muscle and the tendon of the biceps (fig. 102). This needle is directed proximally to reach the anterior aspect of the outer surface of the lateral epicondyle. After contact with bone, 2-4 ml. of lignocaine 0,5-1 % with or without adrenaline are injected while the needle is withdrawn about 0.5 cm. A further 5 ml. should be injected as the point of the needle is drawn back into the subcutaneous tissue. Additional bone contact is made 2-3 times in a direction proximal to the first site of contact and local anaesthetic injected each time (fig. 104). If paraesthesia is elicited, the needle is fixed and 5 ml are injected. If the block is supplemented by a subcutaneous ring of local anaesthetic solution extending from the biceps muscle to the proximal part of the brachioradialis, a block of the superficial branches of the musculocutaneous nerve will result.

INDICATIONS

Surgery of the lower arm and hand in the area supplied by the radial nerve and as a complement to other blocks in the region of the elbow.

As a supplement to axillary brachial plexus block in cases of incomplete anaesthesia of the radial and musculocutaneous nerves.

CONTRAINDICATIONS

Lesions of the nerve are a relative contra-indication.

Nerve Block
at the Wrist

Bertil Löfström

Partial or complete wrist block is of great value for minor surgery. It is particularly valuable in cases where it is desirable to retain some motor function during surgery. N.B. An Esmarch bandage is tolerated only for short periods.

The Median Nerve

ANATOMY

In the forearm, the *median nerve* runs down between the superficial and deep flexors and their tendons. At the level of the proximal crease it comes to lie superficially on the anterior aspect of the wrist, underneath or immediately radial to the tendon of palmaris longus or, should this be missing, between the flexor tendons and the tendon of flexor carpi radialis (fig. 106). The median nerve innervates the palmar surface on the radial side to the midline of the ring finger (fig. 105).

TECHNIQUE

A fine needle (S.W.G. 26-27) is inserted between the tendons of flexor palmaris longus and flexor carpi radialis muscles, at right angles to the skin and at the level of the proximal crease on the wrist. It is an advantage if the hand is dorsiflexed by placing a small rolled-up towel under the dorsal aspect of the wrist. The needle is moved fanwise up and down in a plane at right angles to the long axis of the forearm to obtain paraesthesia. When this is elicited 2-5 ml. of 1 % lignocaine with or without adrenaline are injected slowly (fig. 107) and 2 ml. subcutaneously.

Fig. 106

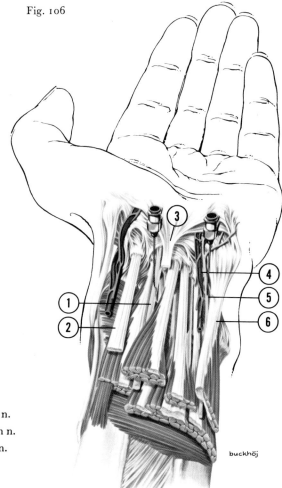

Fig. 105

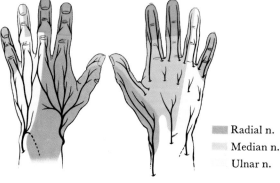

Radial n.
Median n.
Ulnar n.

buckhöj

Carpal tunnel syndrome is a relative contra-indication.

The Ulnar Nerve

ANATOMY

The *ulnar nerve* runs down in the flexor compartment of the forearm, first covered by flexor carpi ulnaris, then passing radial to this muscle (fig. 106). The ulnar artery accompanies the nerve radially. In the distal third of the forearm, approximately 5 cm. proximal to the wrist, the ulnar nerve divides into a *dorsal and palmar branch*. The for-

mer, which is entirely sensory, proceeds beneath the tendon of flexor carpi ulnaris, and thus reaches the dorsal aspect of the wrist, giving branches to the ulnar side of the dorsum of the hand. The palmar branch of the nerve, *r. palmaris n. ulnaris*, which is a mixed nerve, continues along the tendon of flexor carpi ulnaris to divide on the radial side of the pisiform bone into a superficial and a deep branch. The former, which is entirely sensory, is distributed to the ulnar side of the palmar aspect of the hand and to the palmar surfaces of the little finger and the ulnar side of the ring finger (fig. 105).

TECHNIQUE

The palmar branch of the ulnar nerve is blocked on a level with the styloid process of the ulnar. A fine needle (S.W.G. 26-27) is inserted at right angles to the skin, on the radial side of the tendon of flexor carpi ulnaris and the ulnar side of the ulnar artery (fig. 106, 107). The latter can usually be palpated, especially if the wrist is fixed in extreme flexion. Should paraesthesia be elicited, the needle is held in place and 2-4 ml. lignocaine 1 % with or without adrenaline are injected. Even if paraesthesia is not elicited, satisfactory anaesthesia can usually be obtained by injecting 5-10 ml. 1 % solution, while the point of needle is drawn up from contact with the deep fascia and bone until it lies subcutaneously.

To block the dorsal branch of the ulnar nerve, a ring of local anaesthesia is placed subcutaneously around the ulnar aspect of the wrist from the tendon of flexor carpi ulnaris. Approximately 5 ml. of a 0.5-1 % solution of lignocaine with adrenaline are used.

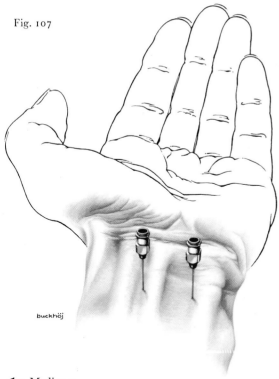

Fig. 107

buckhöj

◀ 1. Median n.
  2. Tendon of the flexor carpi radialis m.
  3. Tendon of the palmaris longus m.
  4. Ulnar a.
  5. Ulnar n.
  6. Tendon of the flexor carpi ulnaris m.

The Radial Nerve

ANATOMY

The superficial branches of *the radial nerve* in the forearm run down, first in company with the radial artery along the medial side of the brachioradialis muscle (fig. 102). About 7 cm. proximal to the wrist the nerve passes underneath the tendon of brachioradialis and lies subcutaneously on the extensor aspect of the lower arm at the level of the wrist. Here it breaks up into several rami, which supply the radial side of the dorsum of the hand (fig. 105).

TECHNIQUE

The superficial ramus can be blocked by infiltrating under the brachioradialis tendon 6-8 cm. proximal to the wrist. However, a simpler and less unpleasant method for the patient is to raise a subcutaneous ring beginning at the level of the tendon of flexor carpi radialis and running round the radial border of the wrist, dorsal to the styloid process of the ulna (fig. 108). Approximately 5 ml. of a 0.5-1.0 % solution of lignocaine with vasoconstrictor are used.

N.B. The ring of infiltration should not extend around the whole circumference of the wrist, and care should be taken not to injure the subcutaneous veins.

Fig. 108

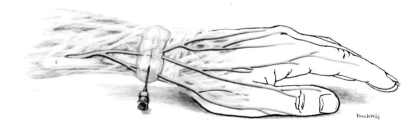

buckhöj

Intercostal Nerve Block

Bertil Löfström

ANATOMY

The *intercostal nerves,* the ventral branches of the mixed thoracic nerves, run segmentally under the respective ribs. Each intercostal nerve, having emerged from its intervertebral foramen, passes through the paravertebral space, separated from the pleura only by the endothoracic fascia. At the costal angle each nerve reaches the caudal margin of the rib and continues below the artery in the costal groove, where it lies between the external and internal intercostal muscle (fig. 109). The upper six intercostal nerves are distributed exclusively to the chest wall, while the lower six continue down to the abdominal wall, where they lie between the internal oblique and transversus abdominis muscles. In the anterior axillary line each intercostal nerve gives off a *lateral cutaneous branch* and near the sternum an *anterior cutaneous branch.* Each cutaneous branch innervates a belt shaped area of skin on the ventro-lateral aspect of the thorax or abdomen (fig. 110) and supplies motor fibres to the intercostal, the transversus thoracis and the abdominal muscles respectively.

Fig. 109

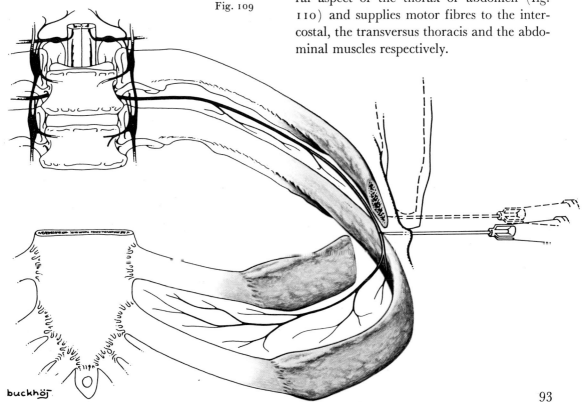

buckhöj

93

For intercostal nerve block the patient may lie either on his side or in the prone position. The latter is preferable should a bilateral block be necessary.

Small doses of thiopentone or other short-acting intravenous anaesthetic may be given immediately before and while the block is being performed. This wille relieve the patient's discomfort and produce optimum working conditions for the anaesthetist (cf. p. 21).

The intercostal nerves can best be blocked in the area of the costal angles, immediately lateral to the lateral border of sacrospinalis muscle. It is easy, as a rule, to palpate the lower ribs. With the arm drawn forwards and upwards the scapula is lifted away from the region of the costal angles, so that it becomes possible to block as far up as the 5th or even the 4th intercostal nerves.

The fingers of one hand palpate the lower margin of the rib and then the overlying skin is drawn up cranially (fig. 111). A fine, 3-5 cm. long needle is inserted towards the rib. The needle should be slightly angulated so that its tip points in a cranial direction. Contact having been made with bone, the needle is slowly moved on the rib until it slips in under the caudal margin of the rib. The needle is then allowed to penetrate to a depth of 3 mm. from the margin of the rib where it is fixed. (N.B. The rib itself is about 7 mm. thick). The needle is moved in and out for 1-2 mm. during the injection of 5 ml. lignocaine 0.5-1 % with adrenaline. For prolonged anaesthesia Moore et al. (1962) recommend amethocaine 0.1-0.25 % with adrenaline 1:200,000 (maximum dose 2 mg. of amethocaine per kg. body weight). The duration of action is 6-8 hours. An analogue of mepivacaine, bupivacaine (0.5 % solution with vasoconstrictor) is claimed to give an even longer duration i.e. about 14 hours (Telivuo, 1963).

The intercostal nerves may also be blocked in the axillary line, should later supplementation of the block be necessary.

For anaesthesia of the abdominal wall blocking of T5-T12 or L1 is required. For lower abdominal surgery an infiltration of the subcutaneous, intramuscular and extraperitoneal tissue just above the anterior superior iliac spine is a useful supplement to intercostal nerve block. For this purpose a 0.5 % solution of lignocaine with a vasoconstrictor is adequate.

INDICATIONS

Fractures of the ribs. A successful intercostal block enables the patient to breath properly, and cough up retained secretions. The analgesia obtained should also be made use of for breathing exercises and physiotherapy.

Fig. 110

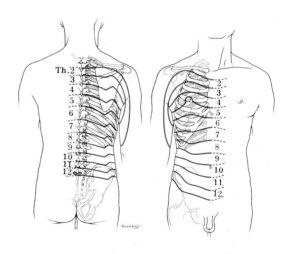

Postoperatively following abdominal surgery to facilitate breathing and coughing.

Intercostal nerve blockade has been and still is used for abdominal surgery as it provides perfect muscular relaxation without the risk of a fall in blood pressure often associated with spinal or epidural anaesthesia. However, in such circumstances coeliac plexus block and/or light general anaesthesia are necessary to permit intra-abdominal manipulations.

COMPLICATIONS

The most important complication is pneumothorax, caused by lung puncture. A pressure pneumothorax may even result. Intercostal blockade must not be attempted, if the rib cannot be palpated with ease. The maximum dose for the local anaesthetic being used should not be exceeded.

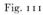

Fig. 111

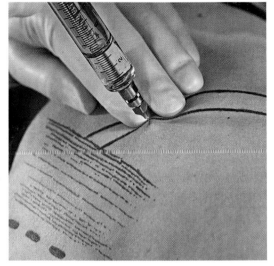

95

Paracervical Block

SÖREN ENGLESSON

SÖREN ENGLESSON

ANATOMY

Pain caused by uterine contractions, the dilatation of the lower uterine segment and of the cervix during the second stage of delivery is mediated by the *sympathetic nerve plexus*. Pain is transmitted from the uterus to the cervix and via the pelvic abdominal sympathetic plexus to the lumbar and lower thoracic segments of the sympathetic chain. Finally the impulses reach the spinal cord by way of *rami communicantes* and the dorsal roots of T11 and T12.

TECHNIQUE

As a rule no additional premedication is given apart from what is normally used in obstetrical practice. If extra premedication is absolutely essential, due consideration must be given to the expected time of delivery, and to the condition of the foetus (cf. p. 22).

The patient is placed in the gynaecological position and the vagina and surrounding skin prepared with bactericidal solution.

The block is performed when the cervix has dilated to 3 cm. in a primiparous or 5 cm. in a multiparous patient. It is best to use a needle which is protected by a guide while being inserted – as, for example, a Kobak needle (fig. 112). By means of the index and middle fingers of one hand, the guide is directed into the lateral fornix of the vagina in the 3 o'clock position. At this stage the needle should point cranially, laterally and dorsally. The needle is then advanced through the guide so as to protrude for about 4 mm (fig. 113) and to penentrate the mucous membrane to this depth (fig. 114). Note how near the needle is to the uterine blood vessels. Following careful aspiration 10-15 ml. of lignocaine or prilocaine 0.5 -1 % or 8-10 ml. of bupivacaine 0.125 (-0,25) % are injected. Should the addition of adrenaline be desired, a low concentration should be used e.g. 1:300,000 or 1:400,000 (the 0.5 or 1.0 % standard solution with adrenaline is mixed with plain solution of the same concentration in a proportion of 2:1 or 1:1 respectively).

This block is then repeated on the other side in the 9 o'clock position in relation to the cervix. Some time should be allowed to elapse between the two blocks in order to avoid high initial concentrations of the drug in the blood, which would result from simultaneous rapid absorption from both sides. Prilocaine has a significantly lower systemic toxicity than lignocaine. However, following

Fig. 112

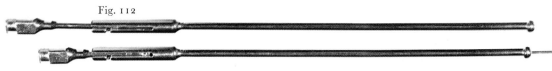

Fig. 113

reinjections of prilocaine the patient should be carefully observed for possible signs of cyanosis due to methaemoglobinaemia (p. 18).

INDICATIONS

Analgesia during the first stage of labour and, in combination with pudendal block during expulsion, the second and third stages of labour as well. When combined with a pudendal block, for the application of a vacuum extractor or mid-forceps. N.B. If paracervical and pudendal block are performed at relatively short intervals strict obervation of the maximum dose of the local anaesthetic agent employed is essential.

Dilatation of the cervix and curettage.

COMPLICATIONS

Too rapid absorption from the loose parametrial tissue can result in high serum concentrations of the drug and generalized toxic symptoms. These should be treated with artificial ventilation with oxygen and control of convulsions with succinyl choline. As this is usually adequate, barbiturate administration should be avoided due to the increased risk of foetal depression.

Note that labour may be prolonged and that the foetus may be depressed if adrenaline is added to the local anaesthetic. Also note the proximity of the uterine artery and vein; thus there is also the risk of direct intravascular injection.

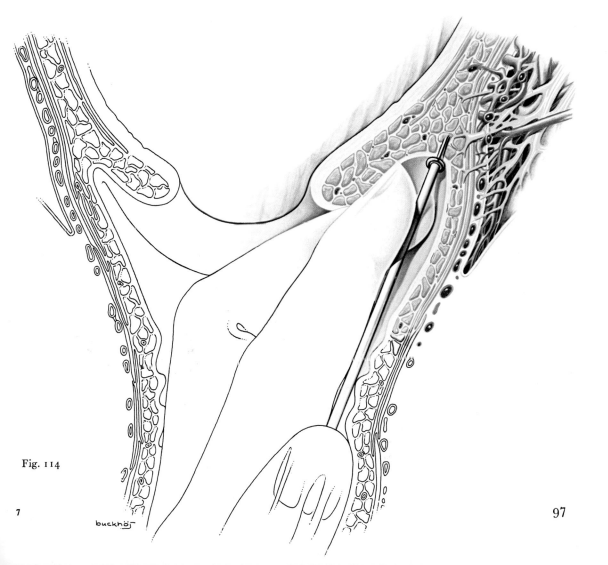

Fig. 114

buckhöj

Pudendal Nerve Block

Sören Englesson

ANATOMY

The *pudendal nerve* (S2, S3 and S4), the chief sensory nerve of the perineum, runs lateral and dorsal to the ischial spine and the sacrospinalis ligament. After passing these structures, it divides into *perineal and inferior rectal nerves* (fig. 115). The perianal part of the perineum and the lower part of the labiae also receive their cutaneous nerve supply from the *perineal rami* which are branches of the *posterior cutaneous nerve of the thigh*. The upper part of the labiae is in addition supplied by the *genito-femoral and ilio-inguinal nerves*.

The pudendal nerve is blocked most conveniently as it passes the ischial spine. Either of two approaches may be used, i.e. the transvaginal route or the perineal route.

TRANSVAGINAL ROUTE

For this route a special long needle, preferably equipped with a guide such as the Kobak needle, should be used (fig. 112, 113).

The patient lies supine with her knees drawn up and well separated, the feet being supported. The perineum and the vagina are swabbed with bactericidal solution. The index and middle fingers of one hand are inserted into the vagina. The ischial spine and the sacraspinous ligament are palpated (fig. 116). The special needle with its point within the guide is inserted and placed on the ligament immediately beside the ischial spine. Then the needle is pushed forward through its guide to pierce the mucous membrane and the ligament (fig. 115), which will produce a popping sensation. The point of the needle should now lie barcly 10 mm from the mu-

Fig. 115

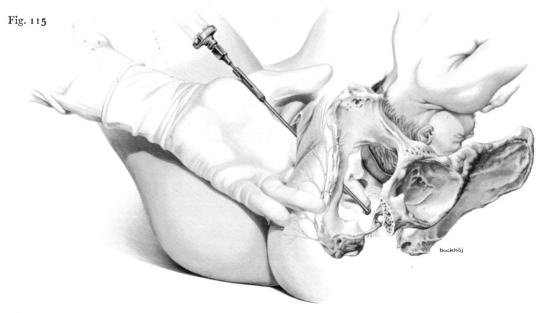

cous membrane and here 10 ml. lignocaine or prilocaine 1 % are injected. The adrenaline content must not exceed 1:200,000. Note that the pudendal artery and vein run parallel to the nerve, so aspiration should be carried out after the injection of every two ml. of solution. If blood has been aspirated, the point of the needle must be moved until no further blood comes back into the syringe. These safety precautions are greatly facilitated by using a syringe with finger rings on both barrel and plunger (e.g. Luer Control Syringe). The procedure is repeated for the opposite nerve.

PERINEAL ROUTE

The perineal route has the advantage that branches of the pudendal nerve and the posterior cutaneous nerve of the thigh can be blocked from the same site of injection (fig. 117). This is necessary both for long oblique episiotomies and for those in the midline.

The patient is placed in position and prepared as for the vaginal approach. With the

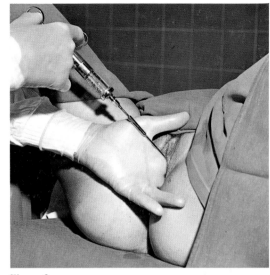

Fig. 116

Fig. 117

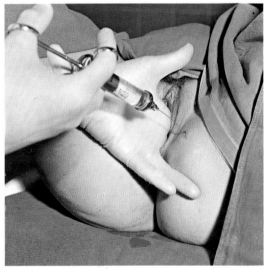

Fig. 118

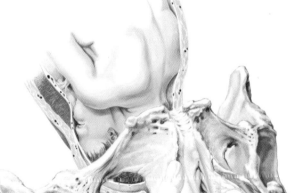

buckhöj

99

index finger of one hand the ischial spine is palpated either rectally or per vaginam. Halfway between the dorsal commissure of the vagina and the ischial tuberosity, a skin weal is raised with a fine-gauge needle. Then a 21 S.W.G. needle, 80 to 120 mm. in length is attached to a 10 ml. syringe and inserted through the weal. With the help of the index finger the tip of the needle is guided towards the ischial tuberosity. Then 5-10 ml. of lignocaine or prilocaine with adrenaline are injected over the lateral and anal aspects of the ischial tuberosity. This results in a block of both the pudendal nerve and the branches of the posterior cutaneous nerve of the thigh. The adrenaline concentration must not exceed 1:200,000.

The syringe is now refilled and 5 ml. of anaesthetic solution injected medial to the ischial tuberosity whilst the needle is inserted into the ischiorectal fossa. The needle is guided dorsolaterally to the sacro-spinous ligament, which is perforated. When the tip of the needle has penetrated 1 cm beyond the ligament 5 ml. of anaesthetic solution are injected (fig. 118). Bilateral block is completed by adopting the same procedure for the other side.

Here too intravascular injection is a constant risk so that repeated aspiration is essential.

For complete anaesthesia of the whole perineum it is necessary to infiltrate subcutaneously along the lateral margins of the vulva and extending right up to the mons pubis (fig. 119). A 0.5 % solution with adrenaline is adequate for this purpose.

INDICATIONS

Pain relief during the second stage of labour, when the vagina, vulva and perineum are being traversed. Low forceps delivery. Episotomy, and suturing of perineal tears. If paracervical block is carried out as well, vacuum extraction or mid-forceps delivery. However, in such cases a strict watch must be kept on the amount of local anaesthetic solution employed in order to avoid overdosage.

COMPLICATIONS

Systemic reactions, particularly following intravascular injection. Haematomata in the gluteal region and upper thigh. Perforation of the rectum, when the perineal route is used. Should a rectal perforation be suspected, the needle is removed and the block performed with a new needle.

Fig. 119

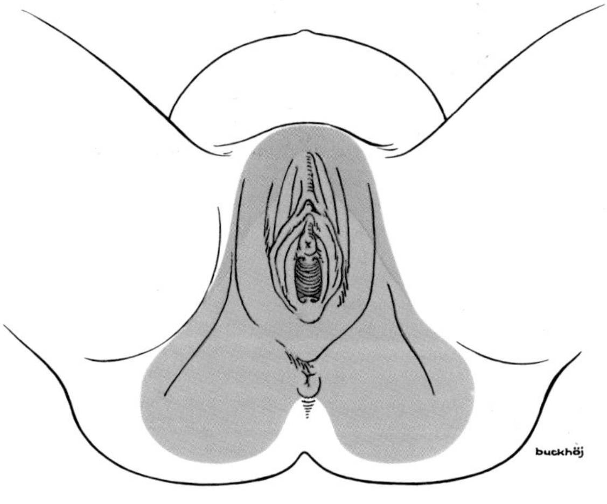

Area supplied by the pudendal nerve
░░ Indeterminate area of mixed innervation (pudendal, ilioinguinal and genitofemoral nn.)
░░ Area of exclusive supply by the pudendal n.

Nerve Block in the Region of the Hip-Joint

BERTIL LÖFSTRÖM (Standard Methods)
SÖREN ENGLESSON (Block of the Sciatic Nerve -Anterior Approach)

Block of the Sciatic Nerve - Posterior Approach

ANATOMY

The sciatic nerve (L4, L5, S1, S2, S3) arises from the *sacral plexus* which lies on the anterior surface of the lateral part of the sacrum. The nerve, which in its upper part is about as thick as a little finger, leaves the pelvis major in company with the *posterior cutaneous nerve of the thigh* and the inferior gluteal artery, through the greater sciatic notch (foramen infrapiriforme) to enter the saddle-area. Covered by the gluteus maximus muscle, the nerve then runs down, dorsal to the gemelli, the obturator internus and quadratus femoris muscles and passes a point approximately equidistant from the ischial tuberosity and the greater trochanter (fig. 120). In continues downwards in the dorsal part of the thigh, where it lies dorsal to the adductor magnus and under cover of the ischiocrural muscles. The sciatic nerve usually divides at the level of the superior apex of the popliteal fossa to form the *tibial* and *the common* peroneal nerves. However, this point of division is often situated more proximally; it can indeed happen that both

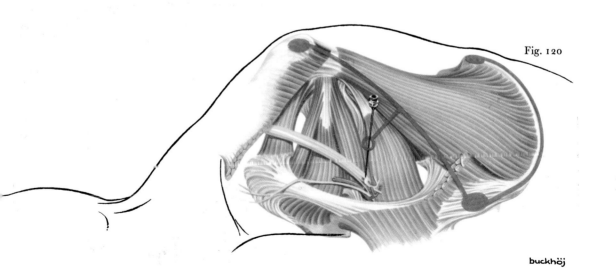

Fig. 120

buckhöj

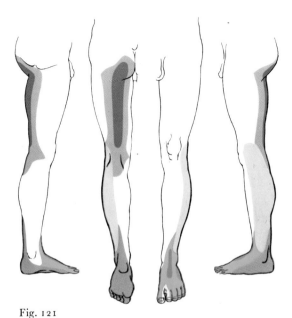

Posterior cutaneous n. of the thigh

Lat. cut. n. of the calf of the
leg (common peroneal n.)

Superficial peroneal n.

Deep peroneal n.

Tibial n.

} sciatic n.

Fig. 121

Fig. 122

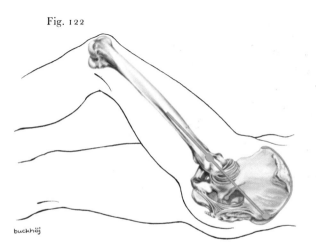

buckhöj

these large branches of the sciatic nerve arise independently from the sacral plexus.

TECHNIQUE

The nerve can be best blocked at its point of exit through the greater sciatic foramen, but it can also be reached at a somewhat more distal point as it passes between the ischial tuberosity and the greater trochanter. However, there appears to be an appreciable incidence of post-anaesthetic ischial pain with nerve block at this latter site. (For block of the sciatic nerve from the anterior aspect of the thigh see page 100).

The patient is placed on the side not to be blocked, tilted half-forward and with the knee bent. A mark is made on the skin overlying the dorsal tip of the greater trochanter, which is equivalent to the point of insertion of the piriformis muscle and another mark is made on the skin overlying the posterior superior iliac spine. A line is drawn joining these two points. The degree of flexion of the hip is adjusted so that the long axis of the femur forms a continuation of this line (fig. 122). In cases of malleolar fracture, for example, it is often simplest to arrange a sup-

Fig. 123

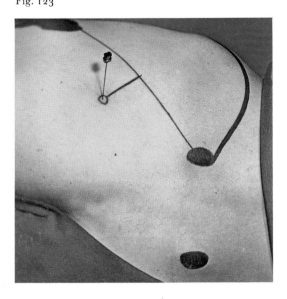

port for the leg below the knee in the position described. From the mid-point of the line drawn between the greater trochanter and the posterior superior iliac spine, a line is drawn at right angles, running caudally and medially. The surface marking of the point where the sciatic nerve emerges from the greater sciatic foramen is situated on this latter line, 4-5 cm. from its intersection with the former line. This point is marked (fig. 123).

Following subcutaneous and intramuscular infiltration, a fine-gauge needle, 10-14 cm. in length with a marker (e.g. the rubber membrane from a Gordh-needle) inserted at right angles to the skin. Contact should be made with bone on or beside the ischial spine. When contact has been made with bone, the rubber membrane is moved down to a point one centimetre from the skin. Since the ischial nerve runs dorsal to the ischial spine the nerve is usually met with before bone. Paraesthesia must be elicited if a high success rate is to be attained. Therefore the anaesthetist endeavours to elicit paraesthesia by inserting and withdrawing the needle in a plane at right angles to the assumed course of the nerve.

The anaesthetist can usually feel when the point of the needle enters the nerve. It feels as if "a fork is inserted into the upper softer part of an asparagus stalk". When paraesthesia has been elicited, 15-30 ml. of 1 % lignocaine with adrenaline are injected slowly. Should paraesthesia be experienced during injection, 5-10 ml. are injected initially, after which the needle is withdawn a few millimetres and a further 10-25 ml. are injected. If complete muscle relaxation is required, 15-25 ml. of a 1.5-2 % solution of lignocaine should be used.

A complete block of the sciatic nerve should be obtained within approximately 30 minutes. This usually extends to the posterior cutaneous nerve of the thigh as well. The extent of the sensory block may be seen from fig. 121.

When sciatic nerve block is performed it must always be borne in mind that the point of the needle traverses a highly vascular area (the inferior gluteal artery and vein, as well as the internal pudendal artery and vein as they pass round the ischial spine). Therefore careful and repeated aspiration is essential.

INDICATIONS

Sciatic nerve block may be used with advantage with malleolar fractures and other fractures below the knee. A disadvantage, however, in such cases is the difficulty in positioning the patient correctly. A sciatic nerve block is not, in general, adequate for reduction of malleolar fractures as the saphenous nerve (a branch of the femoral nerve) usually reaches down to the medial malleolus. However, this nerve can be anaesthetised easily by a subcutaneous injection around the great saphenous vein, medial to the knee joint, or in the lower part of the leg (p. 111, 115).

This type of block is very satisfactory for repair of tendons in the area of the foot and ankle, but is of less value when a bloodless field is required, even when it is combined with femoral nerve block. The patient soon complains of discomfort from the tourniquet or ischaemic pain.

Sciatic and femoral nerve blocks, possibly combined with an obturator nerve block, may also be used prior to reduction of a fracture of the femur. N.B. With such a combined block there is a considerable risk of overdosage.

Sciatic nerve block has been shown to be of great value in minimising the pain from a fractured tibia during transport.

Diagnosis and treatment of neuralgia of the sciatic nerve.

Block of the Sciatic Nerve--Anterior Approach

ANATOMY

After emerging from the greater sciatic foramen (foramen infrapiriforme), the nerve comes to lie between the ischial tuberosity and the greater trochanter, where it is covered anteriorly by the quadratus femoris as well as by the iliopsoas, rectus femoris and sartorius muscles. When the anterior approach to the sciatic nerve is used, the needle passes lateral to the sartorius, and medial to the rectus femoris, and reaches *the sciatic nerve* immediately below the lesser trochanter.

TECHNIQUE

The patient lies supine and the groin and anterior surface of the upper half of the thigh are prepared with antiseptic solution. A line joining the anterior superior iliac spine and the pubic tubercle, which corresponds to the extension of the inguinal ligament is divided into three equal sections (fig. 125). At the point dividing its medial from its middle section a second line is then drawn at right

angles which intersects the original line. The greater trochanter is palpated and a further line is drawn from it parallel to the inguinal ligament. This line intersects the line drawn at right angles and this is the point suitable for insertion (fig. 125) of the needle.

A skin-weal is raised, using a fine needle. A long needle (0.8×120 mm.) is then inserted through the weal and directed slightly laterally, until contact is made with the anterior surface of the femur (fig. 124). The needle is then drawn back as far as the subcutaneous tissue, and redirected so that it passes immediately medial to the femur. The needle is now inserted approximately 5 cm.

Fig. 124

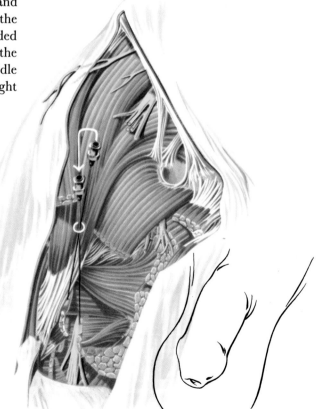

buckhöj

deeper than before, i.e. 5 cm. in excess of the depth required to contact the femur. The needle will now lie ± 1 cm. from the nerve. (fig. 124, 126). A 10 cm. syringe is now attached to the needle and following aspiration the injection of local anaesthetic is started. Should the resistance to injection be very slight, 15-30 ml. of prilocaine or lignocaine 1 %, with adrenaline, is administered. However, if there is appreciable resistance to injection, the point of the needle is moved up and down until the site of least resistance to injection is reached. While this is being sought for, only small quantities should be injected, lest artificial pockets be created, leading later to the mistaken sensation of low resistance. Paraesthesia is not sought for, but is made use of should it occur. The latency is 20-40 minutes. The patient should be prepared in such a way that a femoral block may be performed at the same time (see p. 106).

(see p. 106)

INDICATIONS

Surgery within the area of distribution of the sciatic nerve. The block can be performed without moving the patient onto his side, which is an advantage, especially with painful fractures. This block is usually combined with a femoral block. Thus both skeletal and vascular surgery can be performed on the lower limb. This combination is especially valuable in accident surgery with multiple injuries and in cases of shock where general anaesthesia or a block extending higher up is considered less suitable. This block does not include the groin and supplementary infiltration is required for surgery in that region, e.g. operations for varicose veins.

The maximum dose of the local anaesthetic solution being used must be taken into account to avoid overdosage when a combined sciatic and femoral block is administered.

CONTRAINDICATIONS

In patients suffering from organic nervous disease or painful conditions in the area of distribution of the sciatic nerve, such cases must be assessed on their respective merits.

Skin infection at the site of injection, haematomata or osteomyelitis of the femur or in the track of the needle are contraindications.

Fig. 125

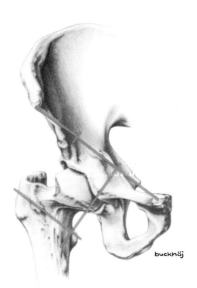

buckhöj

Fig. 126

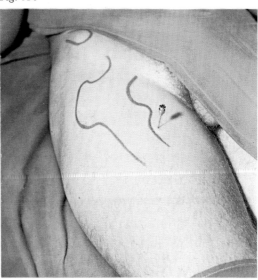

Femoral Nerve Block

ANATOMY

The femoral nerve (L2, L3, L4) runs down from *the lumbar plexus* in the groove between the psoas major and iliac muscles, and enters the anterior part of the thigh by passing deep to the inguinal ligament when it comes to lie anterior to the iliopsoas muscle and somewhat lateral to the femoral artery. Immediately below the ligament, or sometimes even above it, the nerve divides up into two brush-like bundles – an anterior and a posterior group (fig. 127). The anterior branches innervate the skin covering the anterior surface of the thigh, along with the sartorius muscle. The posterior group innervates the quadriceps muscles, the knee joint and its medial ligament and gives off *the saphenous nerve*. This nerve, in company with the great saphenous vein, runs down on the medial side of the calf here supplying the skin right down to the medial malleolus (fig. 130).

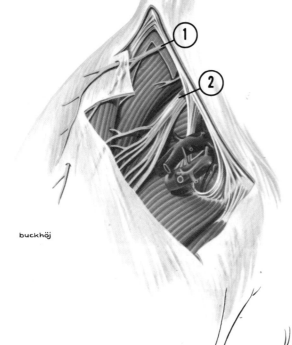

buckhöj

Fig. 127

1. Lateral cutaneous n. of the thigh
2. Femoral n.

The femoral nerve is blocked immediately below the inguinal ligament. The femoral artery is palpated (fig. 128) and a fine relatively short (3-5 cm.) needle is inserted immediately lateral to the vessel to a depth of 3.5-4.0 cm. – i.e. somewhat deeper than the artery. The needle must pulsate when disconnected from the syringe. (Should the artery be punctured, which occasionally happens, arterial compression should be applied for 5-10 minutes to minimise haematoma formation). Approximately 20 ml. of 1 % lignocaine with adrenaline is injected while the needle is moved in and out fanwise from the depth stated and up to the subcutaneous tissue. During this manoeuvre the tip of the needle is gradually moved laterally until it reaches a point approximately 3 cm. from the femoral artery. Paraesthesia is not sought for but should it be obtained, 10 ml. of solution are injected. Nevertheless the fanshaped infiltration described above should always be performed, since in the majority of cases the nerve has already divided at the site of the block.

Fig. 128

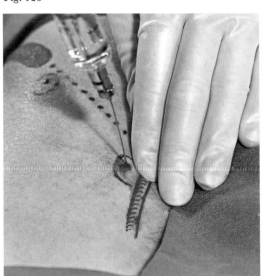

Supplementing a · sciatic nerve block (see pp. 101, 104). *N.B.* There is a certain risk of overdosage with a combined block.

Femoral nerve block, particularly in combination with a block of the lateral cutaneous nerve of the thigh, gives excellent anaesthesia of the anterior aspect of the thigh and its musculature. Operations for varicose veins and of the patella may also be performed under femoral block. For the latter indication the block should be supplemented with a subcutaneous infiltration on each side of the patella. (Suitable for emergency surgery). Diagnosis and treatment of pain.

Block of the Lateral Cutaneous Nerve of the Thigh

ANATOMY

The lateral cutaneous nerve of the thigh (L2, L3) arises from *the lumbar plexus* and runs obliquely downwards and forwards on the inner side of the iliac muscle, to pass deep to the inguinal ligament at a point approximately one finger's breadth medial to the

Fig. 129

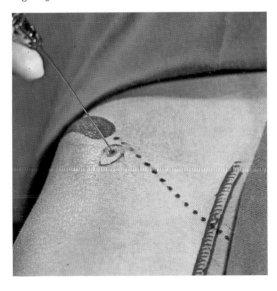

anterior superior iliac spine. It emerges on the lateral side of the thigh, where it lies covered by the fascia lata (fig. 127). Several branches perforate the fascia and supply the skin over the lateral aspect of the thigh (fig. 130).

TECHNIQUE

The nerve is blocked at a point medial to and slightly lower than the anterior superior ilias spine where it lies immediately underneath the fascia lata. A weal is raised 2-3 cm. medial and caudal to the anterior superior iliac spine (fig. 129). A needle 4-5 cm. long is inserted approximately 2 cm. below the anterior superior iliac spine and at right angles to the skin, while 0.5 % lignocaine with adrenaline is being injected. The injections are made fanwise through the fascia lata, directing the needle gradually in a more medial direction. The total volume injected under the fascia lata is 10-15 ml. of lignocaine 0.5 %. As a rule the fascia lata is easily recognised when the point of the needle passes through it.

INDICATIONS

To supplement a sciatic and femoral nerve block respectively. N.B. The administration of such combined blocks carries a certain risk of overdosage.

This block is extremely suitable for anaesthetising the donor area prior to the removal of skin grafts for patients suffering from burns, for example. If a more extensive area of skin is to be removed, it may be combined with a femoral block.

Diagnosis and treatment of neuralgia of the lateral cutaneous nerve of the thigh. The investigation and treatment of pain.

Fig. 130

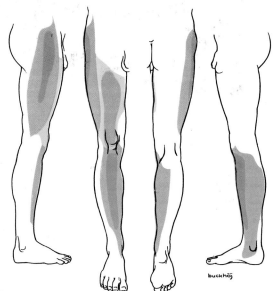

buckhöj

Lateral cutaneous n. of the thigh
Anterior cutaneous branches of the femoral n.
Saphenous n.

108

Obturator Nerve Block

ANATOMY

The obturator nerve (L2, L3, L4), which is a branch of *the lumbar plexus*, appears at the medial border of the psoas muscle on a level with the sacroiliac joint. Covered anteriorly by the external iliac artery and vein, the nerve passes down in the pelvis minor and runs downwards and forwards along its lateral wall to the obturator canal, which it traverses in company with the obturator vessles. It then passes downwards and enters the medial muscular compartment of the thigh. As the nerve passes through the obturator canal, it divides into an anterior and posterior branch (fig. 131). The former supplies the anterior adductor muscles and a cutaneous area on the medial side of the thigh. The size of this area is very variable and often extends down as far as the knee

Fig. 131

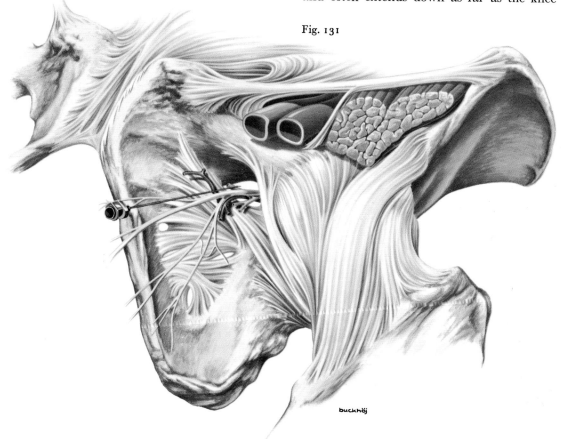

buckhöj

joint. The posterior branch innervates the deep adductor muscles and sends an articular branch to the knee joint (fig. 133).

TECHNIQUE

The pubic tubercle is marked, as well as the other anatomical landmarks in the area, such as the inguinal ligament, the interior superior iliac spine etc. A weal is raised slightly more than 1 cm. below and lateral to the pubic tubercle. While the area is being cleansed with antiseptic solution containing alcohol, the genitalia must be protected to avoid discomfort and smarting. Usually the pubic area must be shaved. Since the needle is to be directed upwards and outwards, it is advisable to cover the area medial to the site of the needles insertion with a sterile drape (fig. 132).

A short fine-gauge needle is inserted at right angles to the skin until its point comes in contact with bone. Lignocaine 0.5 % is injected whilst the needle is advanced. This short needle is then replaced by a 7-8 cm.

long, fine needle which is inserted as far as the pubic bone in the track of the first injection. The position of the needle is then moved so that its point travels laterally and slightly cranially until it enters the obturator canal (fig. 131). When the point of the needle is in the canal, 10 ml. of lignocaine 1 % with adrenaline are injected after careful aspiration. A further 10 ml. are injected as the needle is drawn backwards until it lies subcutaneously.

N.B. Blood vessels accompany the obturator nerve.

A reduction in the power of adduction is indicative of a successful obturator nerve block.

INDICATIONS

Mainly localisation of painful conditions in the hip joint. It is also helpful in the preoperative assessment of a planned transplant of the obturator tendon and, combined with femoral nerve block, for embolectomy (Fogharty catheter technique) (Löfström, to be published).

Fig. 132

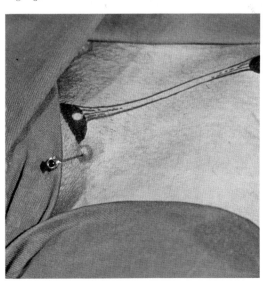

Fig. 133

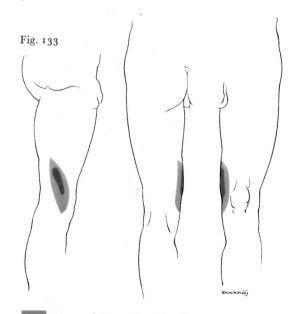

Cutaneous branch of the obturator n.

Nerve Block at the Knee-Joint

Bertil Löfström

In the region of the knee-joint only a block of the saphenous nerve should be attempted, because tibial nerve block is difficult to perform and peroneal nerve block, though simple to carry out where the nerve winds round the head of the fibula, may carry a considerable risk of post-anaesthetic neuritis.

The Saphenous Nerve

ANATOMY

The saphenous nerve, which is the terminal branch of the *femoral nerve,* becomes subcutaneous at the medial side of the knee-joint, immediately below the sartorius muscle. It then accompanies the long saphenous vein right down to the medial malleolus.

TECHNIQUE

The saphenous nerve is blocked by a subcutaneous infiltration in the area of the saphenous vein, immediately below the knee-joint. An injection of 5-10 ml. of lignocaine 0.5 % (−1) % with or without adrenaline is adequate.

N.B. There is a grave risk of intravenous injection in patients suffering from varicose veins.

Nerve Block at the Ankle

Bertil Löfström

The nerves to the foot are relatively easy to block at the ankle. A block at this level, either complete or partial, is a suitable and simple form of anaesthesia for operations on the foot. In the author's experience this has been particularly valuable in cases of diabetic gangrene, when local analgesia will not interfere with the patient's diabetic regime.

The Tibial Nerve

ANATOMY

The *tibial nerve* (L4, L5, S1, S2 and S3), the larger of the two branches of the sciatic nerve, reaches the distal part of the leg from the medial side of the tendo Achilles, where it lies behind the posterior tibial artery and between the tendons of flexor digitorum longus and flexor hallucis longus muscles, covered by the flexor retinaculum (fig. 134). The nerve then gives off the *medial calcaneal branch* to the inside of the heel, after which it divides at the back of the medial malleolus into the *medial* and *lateral plantar nerves*, both of which, under cover of the abductor hallucis, run down to the sole of the foot. The area of skin innervated by this nerve is shown in fig. 136.

TECHNIQUE

The nerve is blocked as it passes behind the medial malleolus. The patient lies prone, his ankles supported by a cylindrical pillow. An area which includes the heel, tendo Achilles and medial malleolus is prepared with bactericidal solution and the anaesthetist endeavours to palpate the posterior tibial artery. A weal is raised slightly lateral to the artery, or, should this be impalpable, immediately to the lateral side of the Achilles tendon at a level with the upper border of the medial malleolus.

A fine-gauge needle, 6-8 cm. long, is inserted at right angles to the posterior aspect of the tibia. The anaesthetist tries to place

Fig. 134

1. Sural n.
2. Short saphenous v.
3. Tibial n.
4. Posterior tibial a.
5. Flexor retinaculum

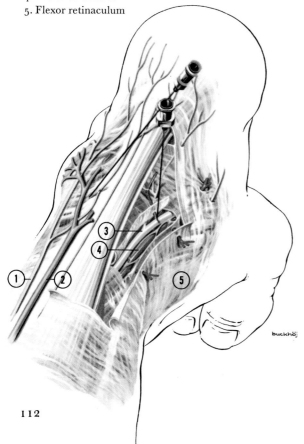

buckhöj

the needle immediately lateral to the posterior tibial artery (fig. 134, 135). If the needle is shifted in a medio-lateral direction, paraesthesia can often be elicited. Should this occur, the needle is held in position and 5-8 ml. lignocaine 0.5-1 %, with or without adrenaline are injected. If paraesthesia is not obtained, 10-12 ml. of solution are injected against the posterior aspect of the tibia while the needle is drawn back 1 cm. This, too, usually provides satisfactory anaesthesia of the plantar surface of the foot. Onset of anaesthesia occurs in 5-10 minutes if paraesthesia has been elicited, but takes up to 30 minutes in its absence.

The area of anaesthesia comprises mainly the sole of the foot, with the exception of its most proximal and lateral parts (fig. 136). It may be supplemented either by block of the sural nerve laterally to the Achilles tendon, or by an infiltration from the calcaneus medially and anteriorly around the medial malleolus.

The Sural Nerve

ANATOMY

The sural nerve is a cutaneous nerve which arises through the union of a branch from *the tibial nerve* and one from *the common peroneal nerve*. It becomes subcutaneous somewhat distal to the middle of the leg and proceeds along with the short saphenous vein behind and below the lateral malleolus, to supply the outer margin of the foot (fig. 134). The area of skin supplied by this nerve is shown in fig. 136.

TECHNIQUE

The sural nerve is blocked by means of a subcutaneous infiltration stretching from the Achilles tendon to the outer border of the lateral malleolus. This is usually performed at the same time as a tibial nerve block by inserting a fine needle lateral to the Achilles tendon and symmetrical with the needle used to block the tibial nerve (fig. 134, 135). Here 5-8 ml. lignocaine 0.5 % with adrenaline are injected whilst the needle is moved fan-wise, within the subcutaneous tissue, between the lateral malleolus and the Achilles tendon.

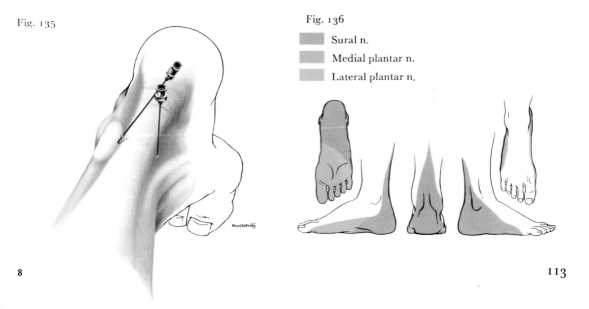

Fig. 135

Fig. 136

■ Sural n.

■ Medial plantar n.

■ Lateral plantar n.

buckhöj

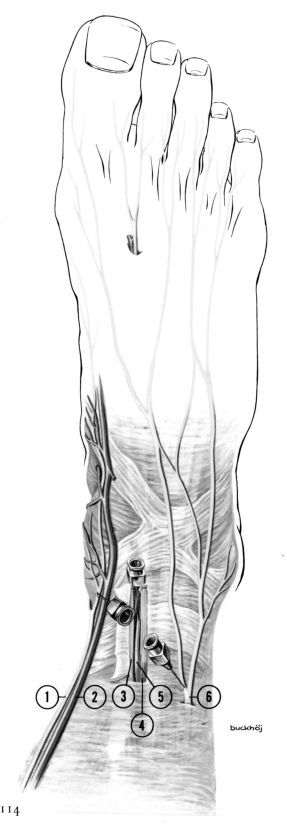

buckhöj

The Superficial Peroneal Nerve, the Deep Peroneal Nerve and the Saphenous Nerve

ANATOMY

The superficial peroneal nerve (L4, L5, S1, S2) perforates the crural fascia on the anterior aspect of the distal two thirds of the leg, and runs subcutaneously down to the dorsum of the foot. (Fig. 137). Its area of distribution to the skin is apparent from fig. 138.

The deep peroneal nerve (L4, L5, S1, S2) runs downwards on the anterior aspect of the interosseus membrane of the leg, lying between the anterior tibial muscle and the extensor hallucis longus muscle (fig. 137). It then continues on to the dorsum of the foot, covered by the superior and the inferior extensor retinaculum. Here it innervates the short extensors of the toes, as well as the skin on the lateral side of the hallux and on the medial side of the second digit. In its course through the anterior muscular compartment of the leg, the nerve lies lateral to the anterior tibial artery. However, distally the nerve crosses under the artery, and so comes to lie medial to it. At the level of the extensor retinaculum, both the nerve and the artery are crossed over by the tendon of the extensor hallucis longus muscle, which runs in a medial direction. Thus when *the deep peroneal nerve* reaches the foot the anterior tibial artery lies lateral to it and the tendon of extensor hallucis longus muscle is on its medial aspect. The cutaneous distribution of *the deep peroneal nerve* is illustrated in fig. 138.

Fig. 137
1. Saphenous n.
2. Long saphenous v.
3. Anterior tibial m.
4. Extensor hallucis longus m.
5. Deep peroneal n.
6. Superficial peroneal n.

The saphenous nerve, which is the sensory terminal branch of *the femoral nerve*, becomes subcutaneous at the lateral side of the knee joint. It then follows the great saphenous vein to the medial malleolus. Its cutaneous distribution is illustrated in fig. 138.

TECHNIQUE

The superficial peroneal nerve is blocked immediately above the talocrural joint. A subcutaneous weal of the local anaesthetic solution is spread extending from the anterior border of the tibia to the lateral malleolus (fig. 137, 139). For this 5-10 ml. of lignocaine 0.5-1 % are required.

The deep peroneal nerve is blocked in the lower part of the leg by inserting the needle towards the tibia, between the tendons of the anterior tibial and the extensor hallucis longus muscles (fig. 137, 139). Here 5-10 ml. lignocaine 0.5-1 % with adrenaline are injected.

The saphenous nerve is blocked by means of subcutaneous infiltration around the great saphenous vein, immediately above the medial malleolus. (Fig. 137, 138). For this 5-10 ml. lignocaine 0.5-1 % with or without adrenaline are adequate. There is a risk of accidental intravenous injection. Hence aspiration is essential.

GENERAL REMARKS

In patients suffering from vascular disease local anaesthetic solutions without an added vasoconstrictor should be used. Plain solutions of mepivacaine or prilocaine give anaesthesia of sufficient duration for operations taking up to 1-2 hours to be performed on the foot or toes.

The injection of a complete ring of local anaesthetic solution around the limb should always be avoided. If this should be required the subcutaneous injections should be performed at different levels. Thus the saphenous nerve may be blocked at the level of the knee (see p. 111).

Fig. 138

▓ Saphenous n.

▒ Superficial peroneal n.

░ Deep peroneal n.

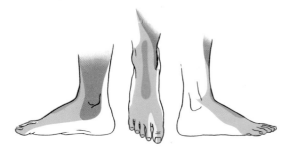

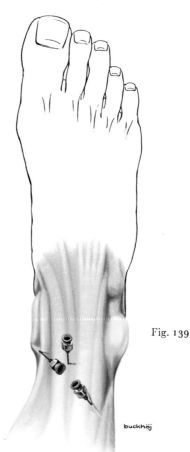

Fig. 139

buckhöj

Spinal Anaesthesia

Torsten Gordh

The injection of local anaesthetic solution into the cerebro-spinal fluid induces a temporary paralysis of the autonomic sensory and motor-nerve fibres in both the anterior and posterior nerve roots which come in contact with the anaesthetic solution.

ANATOMY

Puncture is performed through one of the interspaces between L2 and the sacrum (S1). The spinal cord extends, as a rule, down to L1 or L2. Thus lumbar puncture at or above this region carries the risk of damage to the spinal cord. The most commonly used site for puncture is between L3 and L4. A line drawn between the highest points of the iliac crest usually runs through the spinous process of L4. This line should always be projected onto the skin before a spinal anaesthetic is induced (fig. 140). For teaching purposes it is recommended that the student should palpate and indicate the most important landmarks on the patient's back (fig. 141). These are: A line joining the highest points of the posterior iliac crests, the posterior superior iliac spine, the spine of each lumbar vertebra, the sacrum, with the sacral hiatus, the 12th rib and the spine of the 12th thoracic vertebra which is recognized by a depression on the lower part of the spinous process. The subarachnoid space as a rule extends down to the level of S2. Lumbar puncture prior to spinal anaesthesia should therefore be performed between L2 and S1. The exact site chosen will depend on the extent of anaesthesia required for the proposed operation.

PREPARATIONS

Routine premedication is given, altered as may be required by the patient's general condition and disease. There is a risk of a fall in blood pressure with spinal anaesthesia, especially if a high spinal is given. Therefore a preparatory injection of a vasopressor should be given subcutaneously approximately ½ hour before the administration of the block. The most commonly used agents are ephedrine (50 mg.) or ergotamine tartrate (0.25 mg.) given subcutaneously. Since Klingenström (1960) demonstrated that ergotamine is a valuable prophylactic agent for maintaining blood pressure during spinal anaesthesia, the author has used this drug with great success. A dose of 0.125 mg. (0.5 ml. of a standard solution) is given intravenously and another 0.125 mg. dose subcutaneously just before spinal anaesthesia is produced. The intravenous needle should be left in situ, so that further intravenous injections, or intravenous fluids, may be given, should they be required. Otherwise the patient is prepared in the same way as for general anaesthesia. Careful records are kept just as for general anaesthesia, including initial values of blood pressure and pulse rate. These should then be repeated at 5 minute intervals.

EQUIPMENT

At the Karolinska Hospital, Stockholm, the standard equipment used for spinal anaesthesia consists of: Antoni and Sise needles, wide-bore needle for drawing up solutions, a 2 ml. syringe and a "heavy" solution of the local anaesthetic agent to be employed in a 2 ml. ampoule, ready for subarachnoid injection.

The Antoni (1948) needle is very fine, 10 cm. long and less than 0,5 mm. in diameter. Since the needle is far too flexible to pierce the skin and the interspinous ligament, a Sise introducer is used, through which the Antoni needle is inserted (fig. 142).

Local Anaesthetic Agents: The commonly used local anaesthetic agents may also be used for subarachnoid administration. The solution may either be *hypobaric* ("light") with a lower specific gravity than cerebrospinal fluid, *isobaric,* with a specific gravity equal to that of cerebro-spinal fluid, or *hyperbaric* ("heavy"), with a specific gravity higher than that of cerebro-spinal fluid. The modern technique of spinal punctures using very fine needles of less than 0.5 mm. in diameter, has meant that "heavy" solutions are now mainly used, as smaller volumes (1-2 ml.) of solution are required. These hyperbaric solutions have a higher con-

centration than those used for ordinary local anaesthesia: the most usual drugs are lignocaine 5 % and amethocaine 0.5–1 %. The specific gravity of these solutions is maintained around 1.030–1.040 by the addition of glucose, 5–7.5 %. They are available in 2 ml. ampoules, ready for intrathecal administration, e.g. either lignocaine (100 mg. per ampoule) or amethocaine (20 mg. per ampoule). Re-autoclaving of these solutions should be avoided due to the risk of caramelisation of the glucose content (yellowish-brownish discoloration).

The induction time and duration of anaesthesia depends upon the drug being used. With lignocaine the induction time is about three minutes; with amethocaine it is rather longer. The duration of anaesthesia varies for different anaesthetic agents and for each agent with the level of anaesthesia used as criterion. Thus in the highest segments, where anaesthesia has the shortest duration, lignocaine lasts for approximately 1 hour, prilo-

Fig. 140

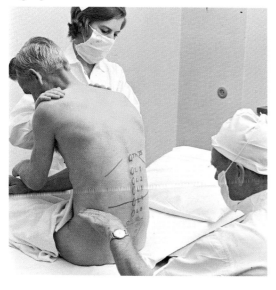

Fig. 141

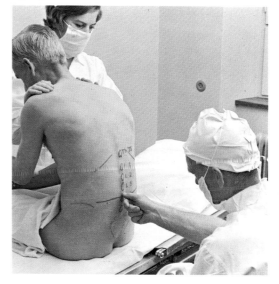

caine approximately 1½ hours and amethocaine approximately 2 hours.

SPREAD OF SPINAL ANAESTHESIA

The extent of anaesthesia following spinal
administration depends mainly on the following factors: The dose and concentration of
the anaesthetic drug, the volume injected,
the site of injection, the speed of injection,
the specific gravity of the solution injected,
the position of the patient during and immediately after the injection and the length of
the vertebral column.

The upward spread of anaesthesia will be
greater the larger the quantity injected and
the higher the interspace used, whether the
injection be performed in the sitting or horizontal position. A long back demands a larger dose or a higher site of injection than a
short one, in order to reach the same level
of anaesthesia. In a large-scale investigation,
the distance from the 7th cervical vertebra
to the sacral hiatus in adults has been found
to vary between 50-75 cm. The shorter vertebral column containing a smaller quantity of
cerebro-spinal fluid results, in the author's
experience, in a greater upward spread of
anaesthesia. It is important to be aware con-
stantly of these conditions, especially when a
high spinal is considered contraindicated.

Fig. 142

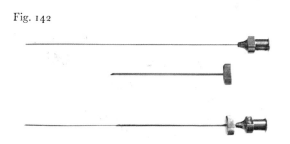

Experience has shown that normal doses
of local anaesthetic result in an unexpected-
ly high level of anaesthesia in patients late
in pregnancy or with large abdominal tumours. Therefore the dosage should be reduced by approximately 50 % and a lower site
of injection should be chosen in such patients.

The spread of the anaesthetic agent is
also influenced greatly by the specific gravity
of the solution and the position of the patient
during and immediately after injection. Following a fixation time of 15-20 minutes the
level of analgesia is usually stabilized and is
not any longer influenced by moving the patient.

Depending on the level of anaesthesia spinal blockade can be divided up into *low spinal, mid-spinal and high spinal anaesthesia.*

LOW SPINAL ANAESTHESIA

A low spinal anaesthesia covers the area of
innervation of *the sacral nerves* (S 1-5) and
as a rule the lower lumbar segment. This
block is adequate for interventions in the perineal and anal regions, the urethra, the outer genitals as well as the vagina and cervix.
Thus low spinal anaesthesia is used for say
cystoscopy, operations for haemorrhoids, operations on the penis and scrotum. However,
low spinal anaesthesia is not adequate for inguinal herniorrhaphy.

The technique described here is somewhat
specialized and demands attention, sensitive
fingers and a certain amount of patience.
Nevertheless it has been used succesfully in
the anaesthetic department at the Karolinska Hospital ever since 1944.

Lumbar puncture and injection are performed with the patient sitting up (fig.
141). The patient is asked to sit up, with his
forearms resting in a relaxed way on his
thighs. The feet are allowed to rest on a low
stool or chair and the patient is then told to

relax completely and lower his head until his chin comes to rest on his chest. At the same time an assistant must support the patient. N.B. With the patient sitting up there is a risk of neurogenic syncope.

Fig. 143

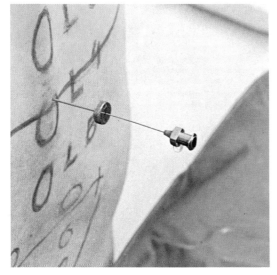

Fig. 144

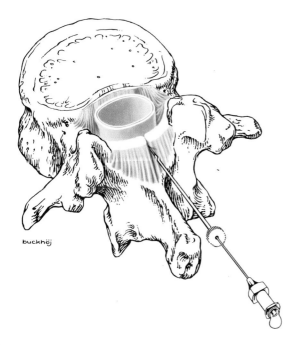

buckhöj

The back is carefully prepared with bactericidal solution. Spinal anaesthesia must be performed under rigorously sterile conditions (with sterile gloves, needless to say). When the anaesthetic solution has been drawn up into the 2 ml. syringe, the Sise introducer is inserted between L4 and L5 or between L5 and S1, in the mid-line and at right angles to the skin. If the needle is sharp enough and the patient has been warned, its rapid introduction in one single movement causes no more pain than the raising of a small intracutaneous bleb with a fine needle. The needle is inserted about 2 cm. through the ligamentum flavum. The Antoni needle is now inserted through the introducer. A "hanging drop" of anaesthetic solution is supended from the end of the needle (fig. 143, 144). The hub of the needle is grasped by the thumb and index finger of both hands, while the little fingers rest against the patient's back. Meanwhile, the shaft of the needle is supported by the third and fourth digit, again of both hands. Thus the needle is firmly held and supported against the patient's back (fig. 145). The needle is then inserted slow-

Fig. 145

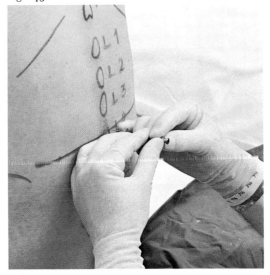

ly and carefully, watching the hanging drop all the time. A slight but definite resistance is felt while the needle is piercing the ligamentum flavum. This disappears as soon as the ligament is pierced and the needle enters the epidural space. Meanwhile, the hanging drop is sucked into the hub of the needle by the negative pressure normally found in the epidural space (fig. 146). This is clearly demonstrable in 80 % of cases. One knows now that only a few millimetres remain before the dura is pierced. By making use of the negative pressure in the epidural space in the same way as during epidural anaesthesia, the anatomical position of the point of the needle is assessed. Thus the needle is not inserted too far and the risk of damaging the nerve roots is minimized. At the same time this technique may provide useful practice in the identification of the epidural space.

The perforation of the dura gives a sensation similar to piercing a stretched piece of parchment and, indeed, it can sometimes be heard. As soon as the dura is pierced, the pressure becomes positive and cerbrospinal fluid begins to drop from the hub of the needle (fig. 147).

Contact with bone during spinal puncture usually indicates that the needle has struck the vertebral lamina. If the needle is forced against bone and periosteum, the lumen of the needle may easily be blocked. If there is reason to suspect that this may have occurred it is wise to take out the Antoni needle, and flush it through with anaesthetic solution. When the direction of the Antoni needle is changed, it must be drawn back completely into the introducer before a fresh attempt is made in a different direction. Thus various angles are tried until bone is no longer met with. With increasing experience one acquires a sort of "anatomical touch" of the depth required for the puncture considering the thickness of the soft tissue between skin and ligamentum flavum. If the point of the needle is considered to lie in the subarachnoid space, about 0.1 ml. of anaesthetic solution may be injected to rinse the needle. This often causes the C.S.F. to flow back into the needle.

Fig. 146

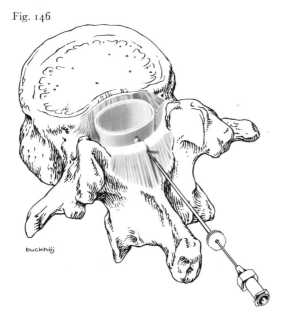

Fig. 147

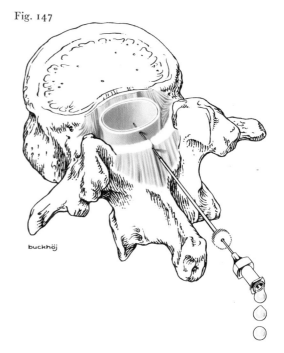

Should the mid-line approach prove unsuccessful the *lateral approach* may be tried. The introducer is inserted 1.5 cm. from the mid-line at the level of the interspace and is directed at an angle of 25° towards the mid-line. The needle will then come to lie lateral to the interspinous and supraspinous ligaments. With this technique, too, several attempts may have to be made in various directions – both upwards and downwards, until the ligamentum flavum is found.

Blood appearing at the hub of the needle may mean that the point of the needle has pierced a blood vessel. In this case the drops of C.S.F. will soon become clearer and the blood will lie as a sediment in the drops. However, injection is not carried out until the C.S.F. is quite clear. Should the C.S.F. remain mixed with blood, an intradural haemorrhage may be suspected. If this happens it is wise to cancel the procedure and if possible postpone the operation. Bleeding can be increased by a general anaesthetic associated with straining.

When the dura is pierced and a clear drip of cerebrospinal fluid from the needle is obtained, 1 ml. of anaesthetic solution is injected. After this, the Antoni and Sise needles are rapidly withdrawn. During injection it is recommended that the needle be held as shown in fig. 148. With the dorsal surface of the hand resting against the patient's back while the needle and syringe are firmly held, the risk of displacing the needle is reduced, even if the patient should move.

The patient is now asked to sit for one or two minutes, to allow the heavy solution to sink down in the subarachnoid space and thus block the sacral roots. The patient is then turned onto his back, with his head slightly raised.

MID-SPINAL ANAESTHESIA

This is used for operations below the level of *the umbilicus* (T10), such as appendicectomy, prostatectomy, herniorrhaphy, gynaecological operations and operations on the lower limbs.

The *technique* and equipment are the same as for a low spinal. The injection is

Fig. 148

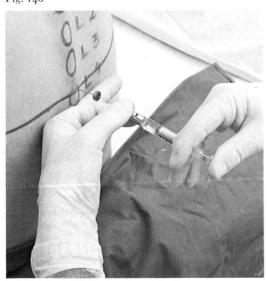

Fig. 149

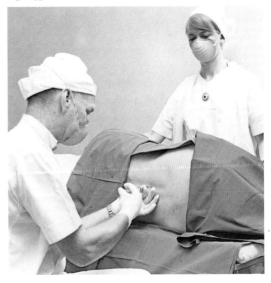

performed with the patient either sitting, or lying on his side.

Injection in the sitting position is used as a rule for operations on the lower limbs, in which case the interspace between the 3rd and 4th lumbar vertebrae is chosen and 1.0-1.5 ml. of local anaesthetic solution are injected. Thereafter the patient is immediately placed supine. Should the proposed operation be in the inguinal region or higher, the patient lies with a slight (10°) head-down tilt until the level of anaesthesia has reached the height desired. It is most important that the spread of the anaesthetic is checked carefully and frequently. The first symptom of the anaesthetic drug's action on the spinal roots is a sensation of warmth in the feet. A rapid upward spread of anaesthesia now takes place. The primary sensation of warmth is probably due to stimulation of afferent thermal (heat) fibers by the local anaesthesia solution. The effect of sympathetic paralysis occurs later, ca. 5 minutes. (T. Gordh, Regional Anaesthesia 1977, Vol. 2).

The best and most pleasant way to test the *level of anaesthesia* is to use a swab moistened with ether as the loss of temperature and pain sensation proceeds simultaneously. In this way the border between complete anaesthesia and partial loss of sensation is often more reliably defined than by repeated pinpricks, or by pinching the skin with an artery forceps, methods which are, moreover, uncomfortable for the patient. As soon as the desired level of anaesthesia is reached the patient is placed horizontally with the head elevated by a pillow.

With the above technique it is not always possible to produce anaesthesia right up to the level of the umbilicus, as is required for such operations as prostatectomy, appendicetomy, or even inguinal hernioraphy in patients with a long vertebral column.

Injection in the lateral decubitus provides a more reliable level of anaesthesia. The patient lies horizontally on the side on which it is proposed to operate. N.B. Hyperbaric solution. His knees are drawn up and his chin is inclined towards his knees (fig. 149). The maintenance of the best position, one of flexion of the vertebral column, is facilitated if an assistant supports him across his shoulders and behind his knees. Lumbar puncture is performed between L3 and L4 and 1.0-1.5 ml. of anaesthetic solution are injected. After the injection, the patient is turned on to his back. If the level of anaesthesia is to reach the umbilicus an initial slight head-down tilt may be necessary. As previously described, it is now essential to check the spread of anaesthesia frequently and with care. As soon as the patient indicates a slightly reduced sensation of cold when ether comes in contact with the skin at the desired level of anaesthesia the patient is immediately returned to the horizontal position, in order to avoid an unnecessarily high level of anaesthesia.

Lumbar puncture is always easier to perform with the patient sitting up. Should it be difficult in the lateral position, it is permissible to perform the puncture with the patient sitting up; then, with the needle in place, to move him carefully to the lateral position, without moving or rotating his vertebral column – because of the risk of breaking the needle. Should the result of injection be unsatisfactory a new spinal block may be performed. However, in this case a smaller dose is to be given (usually about half the original dose).

HIGH SPINAL ANAESTHESIA

In high spinal anaesthesia the level of anaesthesia is expected to reach the *nipple line* (T4), permitting the performance of operations in the upper abdomen, such at those on the stomach and biliary tract. The indications for high spinal anaesthesia are much fewer since the advent of the muscle relaxants. Complications such as hypotension, hiccup and vomiting during the operation have also reduced its use for upper abdominal surgery.

Technique and equipment are the same as for a mid-spinal anaesthesia in the lateral position. Usually lumbar puncture is performed between L 2 and L 3 and the dose varies between 1.5 and 2 ml. In order to reach the required level of anaesthesia the injection may even have to be performed with the patient in a slight head-down position, especially if he has a long back. The height of anaesthesia reached must be carefully watched, since there is a considerable risk of total spinal anaesthesia, with intercostal paralysis and respiratory insufficiency or even arrest.

INDICATIONS

Spinal anaesthesia provides excellent muscle relaxation and is most suitable for powerfully built, muscular and overweight patients who are difficult to manage under general anaesthesia. Pyknic patients are more suitable for spinal anaesthesia than asthenics. Urological and gynaecological surgery, operations on the lower limbs and other operations below the level of the umbilicus, may well be performed under spinal anaesthesia. It is also suitable for patients suffering from respiratory disease. Spinal anaesthesia has a negligible effect on metabolism and body chemistry. It can therefore be administered to patients suffering from liver and kidney disease, as well as diabetes.

The technique of, and indications for, spinal anaesthesia as practiced in the Department of Anaesthesia, Karolinska Hospital, have been presented. The technique has been described in detail because the author considers careful technique to be essential in order to avoid neurological complications which are most feared by both patient and anaesthetist.

CONTRAINDICATIONS

A patient must never be forced to accept spinal anaesthesia against his will, except for reasons of safety, nor should it be used in children. Spinal anaesthesia is also contraindicated in patients who are in shock or suffer from hypoxia, hypovolaemia, severe anaemia or marked dehydration. High spinals should not be administered to patients who have recently suffered from myocardial infarction, or suffer from coronary ischaemia with high blood pressure, because of the risk of a fall in blood pressure. Furthermore, spinal anaesthesia is contraindicated in patients with active neurological disease, or in those with a history of frequent headache. An absolute contraindication is infection and sepsis near the site of the injection.

COMPLICATIONS

The patient's circulation and ventilation are affected in direct proportion to the height of anaesthesia. Thus from this point of view spinal anaesthesia is to be considered as a general anaesthetic even though only a part of the body is anaesthetized. As a rule, a spinal anaesthetic is fixed within 15-20 minutes; therefore circulatory or respiratory embarrassment should be apparent within this period.

Effect on the Circulation: The most important is *hypotension,* caused by a preganglionic block of the sympathetic fibres in the anterior roots resulting in vasodilatation and a reduction in the venous return to the heart. Treatment consists in tilting the patient head-down, the administration of oxygen and the intravenous administration of a va-

sopressor. Severe hypotension – the so call-
ed "spinal shock" – is a serious complication,
but has become rare since the prophylactic
administration of ergotamine has been introduced. A fall in blood pressure is seldom
seen with a low spinal, since the sympathetic
chain is not involved.

Respiratory Complications: High spinal
anaesthesia is accompanied by a rising intercostal muscle paralysis, and the patient cannot speak, but only whisper. He must be given
oxygen and artificial ventilation, should that
be necessary, until the paralysis has reco-
vered.

Other Complications: Disturbing *hiccup* and
nausea often follow high spinal anaesthesia,
especially in conjunction with vagus stimulation and manipulation of the viscera during
the operation. When requested, or when
dealing with very nervous and anxious patients, spinal anaesthesia may be combined
with a suitable sedative or even light general
anaesthetic e.g. thiopentone or nitrous oxide
and oxygen, before the operation is commenced.

Late Complications of Spinal Anaesthesia:
Headache is seen with this technique in
about 2 % of cases (Franksson & Gordh
1946). The cause is thought to be a fall in
the pressure in the C.S.F. following leakage
through the puncture in the dura. It is usually relieved when the patient lies horizontally and is seldom prolonged. *Meningitis* is
an uncommon complication, which may be
a consequence of inadequate sterile precautions. *Neurological Complications* ranging
from paraplegia to transient paresis and paraesthesia have been described. They are
thought to be caused by local damage, such
as direct mechanical injury to the spinal cord
or nerve roots, arachnoiditis following bleeding, chemical or infectious irritation. These
complications, which competent anaesthetists
very seldom see (Arner 1952) are reduced in frequency when careful lumbar puncture and a strict aseptic technique are used.
Since 1945 about 50,000 spinals have been
performed in the Department of Anaesthesia
at the Karolinska Hospital without any serious neurological complications.

Lumbar Epidural Anaesthesia

Sören Englesson

ANATOMY

The *epidural space* (extradural space, peridural space) is the space between the two layers of the dura mater formed by its division at the edge of the foramen magnum (fig. 150). The outer layer forms the periosterum of the vertebral canal; the inner the actual *dura mater spinalis*. The epidural space is limited caudally by the *sacrococcygeal ligament*. It contains a number of venous plexus as well as fat and connective tissue. In the lumbar vertebral column the spinal canal is triangular in cross-section, with one of the angles lying dorsally. The greatest distance to dura mater lies in the mid-line posteriorly and is 5 mm. on average.

Situated between the vertebrae, and limited laterally by their articular processes, is the interlaminar foramen – the gap between the laminae of adjoining vertebrae. This is ovoid in the lumbar region, but becomes flatter both cranially and caudally, also extending laterally the higher up one goes in the thoracic vertebral column. The interlaminar foramen is covered by the *ligamentum flavum*, which is an important landmark when the epidural space is being approached. The dural sac ends at the middle of the sacral canal, on a level with S 2-S 3; and the spinal cord ends between L 1-L 3. It is recommended – especially for beginners – that epidural puncture be performed in the interspace between L 3-L 4 or L 4-L 5, because the spinal cord does not extend down to this level. Both

Fig. 150

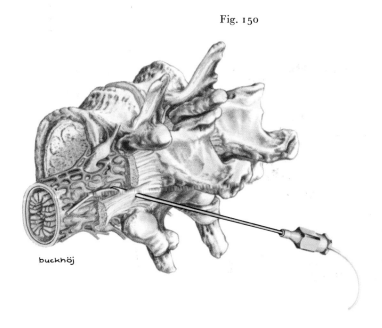

buckhöj

thoracic and cervical epidural puncture may be performed, but these require greater care and experience.

MECHANISM OF ACTION

It is still not certain where the anaesthetic agent acts, but several hypotheses regarding its mechanism have been suggested. According to one of them the local anaesthetic agent acts in the subarachnoid space following diffusion through the dura. According to another hypothesis the solution may follow the nerves through the intervertebral foramina thus resulting in a paravertebral block. Perhaps the most likely mechanism is that the solution penetrates the dural cuffs and runs subpially along the nerves back to the spinal cord, while simultaneously entering the nerves by diffusion. Here, too, the finest fibres with the least myelin are anaesthetized first – as for example, the sympathetic nerve fibres, – while nerve fibres of greater diameter and containing more myelin – as for example, motor and proprioceptive fibres – are anaesthetized last.

EQUIPMENT

The equipment needed (fig. 151) consists of a sterile split towel, a cup for the anaesthetic solution and a 10 ml. syringe the piston of which moves easily. The syringe should preferably be fitted with suitable finger rings. A 0.6×22 mm. (No. 16) and a 8×80 mm. needle are required for the infiltration of the skin and underlying tissues. Finally epidural needles are necessary. The type recommended here is the Tuohy-Flower needle (17 or 18 gauge, i.e. 1.5 or 1.25 mm. respectively). It has a curved and rather blunt point, to minimize the risk of puncturing the

Fig. 151

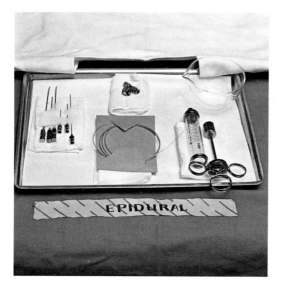

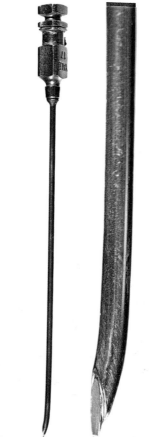

Fig. 152 a   Fig. 152 b

dura (fig. 152 a). This needle is equipped with a stilette, longer than the needle and sharpened to facilitate its passage through the skin and underlying tissue (fig. 152 b). For continuous epidural anaesthesia, catheters of polyvinyl are required which are marked from one end in 5 cm. graduations up to 15 cm. Preferably each catheter should be equipped with an introducer of piano-wire and an adapter which fixes it by means of a rubber chuck. Naturally, there are other catheters as well, with or without this special adapter.

IDENTIFICATION OF THE EPIDURAL SPACE

The identification of the epidural space may be performed in various ways.

The loss-of-resistance technique is perhaps the most frequently employed. It relies on the fact that there is marked resistance to injection through the epidural needle as long as its point lies in the ligamentum flavum. When the needle enters the epidural space this resistance disappears almost completely. There are many indicators, such as syringes with spring-loaded pistons or a small air-filled balloon attached to a Luer or Record adapter (Macintosh balloon) which purport to assist in demonstrating this loss of resistance. However, the simplest method is to exert pressure manually on the plunger of a syringe containing local anaesthetic or preferably saline solution attached to the needle. Naturally, only syringes whose plungers move freely are suitable for this purpose.

The hanging drop technique consists in placing a drop of anaesthetic solution on the hub of the needle, when its point is in the ligamentum flavum. The needle is then pushed carefully forward. When the needle enters the epidural space, this drop is suddenly sucked into the needle, due to the negative pressure which is usually present in the epidural space. This method is not completely reliable, since this negative pressure may disappear for various reasons, for example, with forced expiration or breathholding.

POSITION

During puncture the patient may be sitting or lying in the lateral position. In both cases the back and the neck should be flexed in order to open up the interspinous spaces and facilitate entry of the needle. If the patient is lying on the side the knees should be drawn up, while in the sitting position the feet should rest on a stool.

Lumbar puncture in the sitting position is practised mainly for low epidural blocks, particularly of the sacral segments. However, for this procedure an assistant is required to keep the patient in the correct position. As a rule lumbar puncture in the lateral position is preferred since this position is much more comfortable for the patient. The back is prepared with bactericidal solution and covered with a drape with a hole in it and the anaesthetist dons sterile gloves. Handling the catheter under sterile precautions is greatly facilitated if the anaesthetist wears a sterile gown.

MEDIAL APPROACH

A skin weal is raised in the interspace chosen for puncture. The Tuohy needle is inserted with its orifice directed cranially in a sagittal plane and pointing slightly cranially, as far as the ligamentum flavum. Here a marked increase in the tissue resistance is experienced. The stilette is now removed and replaced by the syringe containing normal saline or 0.5 % local anaesthetic solution (fig. 153). The needle is advanced slowly and carefully while constant pressure is exerted on the plunger until the entrance into the epidural space is observed by the loss of resistance (fig. 154). In adults the distance from the skin to the epidural space in the lumbar area is between 3 and 5 cm.

It is most important that the hand used to advance the needle rests firmly against the patient's back all the time in order to have maximum control of the movement of the needle and to avoid accidental puncture of the dura. The catheter's introducer is withdrawn 1 cm. from its point, and the catheter is rolled up in one hand. The catheter is fed through the lumen and gently eased past the point of the needle. It is pushed in until the point lies at the desired height – usually 3-5 cm. from the point of the needle. During this manoeuvre the catheter is supported by the introducer and guided by the orifice of the Touhy needle, which faces cranially. Should the insertion of the catheter be obstructed, it must on no account be withdrawn through the needle; both must be removed together, since a piece of the catheter can easily be sheared off. When the catheter is in place the needle is drawn out using one hand, whilst the catheter is fixed with the other. The introducer is removed and the adapter is coupled to the catheter. If the cap is placed on

Fig. 153

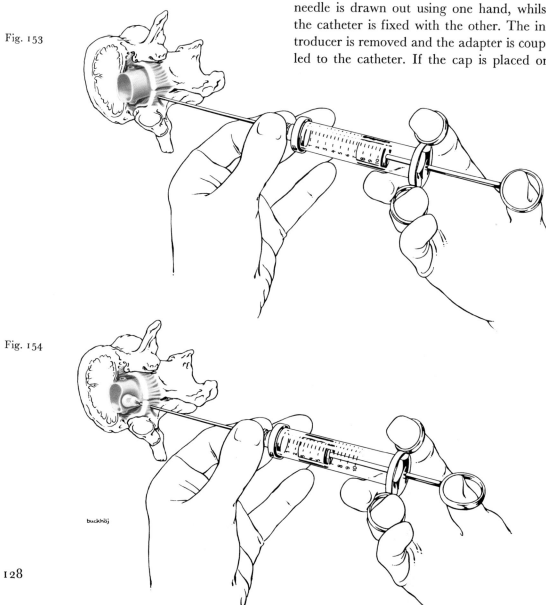

Fig. 154

buckhöj

128

the adapter, the end of the catheter is stopped automatically at the right depth. Provided that neither cerebrospinal fluid nor blood is obtained on aspiration, a test dose of 50-60 mg. lignocaine is administered. (Should the catheter still lie intradurally this dose would produce motor block in the legs. If this were to happen the operation may be performed under spinal anaesthesia). The catheter is fixed loosely with elastoplast along the back up to the shoulder, so that the adapter is accessible for further injections.

LATERAL APPROACH

A skin-weal is raised 1 cm. lateral to the caudal margin of the spinous process. Using a 0.8×80 mm. needle, small quantities of local anaesthetic are injected from this point fanwise until the vertebral arch is reached. The periosteum is anaesthetized (fig. 155). The depth to the bone is noted. The epidural needle is now inserted mainly in a similar direction towards the bone, but making contact with it slightly medially and cranially

to the original point of contact. The needle is now prodded on to the vertebral arch until the point slips off it and into the interlaminar foramen. The point of the needle should be lying near the mid-line. At this stage the stilette is removed and the passage of the needle through the ligamentum flavum into the epidural space is guided by the "loss of resistance test". As above, the back of the hand responsible for the insertion of the needle must rest firmly against the patient's back. The catheter is then inserted as previously described (fig. 156) and following aspiration, the test dose is injected.

The advantage of this method is that the vertebral arch forms a fixed point which facilitates the estimation of the depth to the ligamentum flavum. Furthermore, the needle enters the epidural space at a more oblique angle, which facilitates the insertion of the catheter. Also, the interspinous ligament, which can be calcified in older patients, need not be penetrated. This technique is less dependent upon the patient's ability to separate the spinous processes by flexing his vertebral column.

Fig. 155

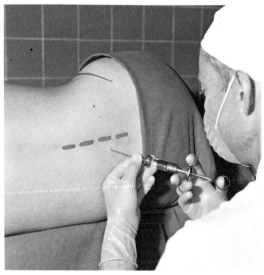

Fig. 156

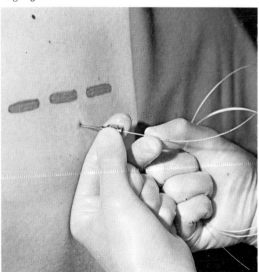

The spread of the local anaesthetic solution deposited into the epidural space proceeds both upwards and downwards from the site of its injection. The position of the trunk is significant since the solution spreads mainly downwards in patients who are sitting up. However, this is not so marked as with spinal anaesthesia when using hyperbaric solutions. The first injection has also a certain tracking effect. Thus a second dose injected through the same catheter is distributed primarily to the same segmental area as the first dose, even if the position of the body has been changed meanwhile. Therefore a second dose after, say, 15-20 minutes in order to increase the area anaesthetized must be at least as large as the first to produce the desired effect. If the second dose is smaller than the first one, a mere deepening of anaesthesia in already anaesthetized segments is obtained.

Following the injection into the epidural space there are considerable losses due to leakage through the intervertebral foramina and also absorption into the systemic circulation. These losses are greatest in the age group 16-20 years, and decrease in a practically linear proportion with increasing age. Therefore the dose required to give a certain level of anaesthesia depends primarily on the age of the patient, and, to a lesser extent, on his height. Changes with age in blood vessels, areolar tissue etc., tend to reduce the size of the epidural space as well as the losses due to reabsorption and leakage from that space. Patients with manifest signs of ageing, e.g. arteriosclerosis and diabetic gangrene, require a significantly smaller dose than a healthy individual of the same age. A woman in the later stages of pregnancy requires a smaller dose than a non-pregnant woman. This may well be due to an increased venous pressure in the lower part of the body caused by the gravid uterus and a subsequently increased volume of blood in the epidural venous plexus, resulting in a decrease of the capacity of the epidural space.

A GUIDE TO DOSAGE

Epidural anaesthesia can be induced either by a single injection directly through the needle, or via a catheter inserted into the epidural space. The former method is in general satisfactory, but the catheter technique increases the possibility of prolonging the period of anaesthesia and increasing its extent should the need arise.

The choice of a suitable dose involves special problems due to individual variations in effect. The following scheme may serve as a guide:

The number of segments to be anaesthetized in order to block the afferent impulses from the operative field is determined (calculating from 5 sacral, 5 lumbar and 12 thoracic segments). The patient's age is noted. According to Bromage (1962) a 20 year old patient requires 1.5 ml. per segment if a 2 % lignocaine solution is used and the injection is made in the lateral position at the level L_2/L_3. If on the other hand the patient is 80 years of age only 0.75 ml. of this solution are needed per segment (fig. 157). The number of ml/segment is read off from the graph and multiplied by the chosen number of segments. The dose is reduced by about $1/3$ in pregnant patients near term and in elderly patients with manifest arteriosclerosis. It should be noted that this applies to a 2 % solution of lignocaine. Should a lower concentration be used, the volume is increased somewhat – but not so much that an equivalent dose of lignocaine in mg. is given.

The concentration to be used is chosen according to the following scheme:

2 % solutions are used when complete muscle relaxation is required, e.g. for abdominal surgery or for reduction of fractures.

1 %-1.5 % solutions may be employed when muscle relaxation is not so important. Should the need for greater muscle relaxation arise during the course of the operation this may be obtained in most cases by a repetition of the same dose which had been given originally. (Lignocaine 2 % and 1 % correspond roughly to bupivacaine 0,5 % and 0.25 % respectively).

If sympathetic fibres alone are to be affected 0.5 % solutions are sufficient. The adrenaline concentration should be kept as low as 1:200,000. A 0.5 % solution may also be used with advantage for continuous epidural anaesthesia during the first stage of delivery. This weak solution has only minimal effect on motor function and the patient can still be made to bear down. For the second stage the depth of analgesia can easily be increased by injecting a 1 % solution (preferably with the patient sitting up).

A preliminary test of the extent of the blockade may be performed about ten minutes after the first injection. Frequently only an approximate idea of the extent and depth of anaesthesia can be obtained so soon after the

administration. This should also be pointed out to the patient. The hypo-algesia or analgesia now present can best be demonstrated by contrast. Thus repeated pinpricks or an ether-swab are applied moving from the anaesthetized area into a less anaesthetized area, e.g. longitudinally at 5 cm. intervals and at a distance of 5 cm. from the midline starting from the groin and up to the nipple line (fig. 158). Usually the patient can state where the intensity of the pinprick increases. From this the boundaries of the area where anaesthesia will be complete 10-20 minutes hence may be mapped out.

INDICATIONS

Lumbar epidural anaesthesia is suitable for all types of surgery below the umbilicus. Adequate premedication augmented by a sedative immediately before the operation commences, possibly combined with small repeated intravenous doses of a short acting barbiturate is often sufficient to provide "twilight sleep", which most patients find very comfortable.

Epidural anaesthesia is especially suitable for patients who wish to be awake during surgery and for younger patients who are more prone to postspinal headache than are older patients. It is indicated for emergency surgery in patients who are liable to vomiting and aspiration; in patients with lung disease where it is considered undesirable to interfere with a balanced ventilatory state, or with infections – for example – open pulmonary tuberculosis.

Obstetric analgesia.

Sympathetic block of the lower part of the body.

For various painful conditions including post-operative pain. In blocks of longer duration, the catheter should be changed every second or third day, to avoid infection.

Fig. 157

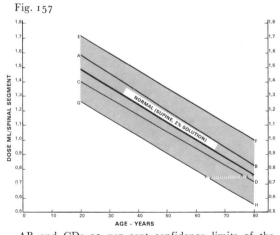

AB and CD: 95 per cent confidence limits of the mean.
EF and GH: 95 per cent of all normal patients fall within these limits.

Inadequately treated haemorrhagic shock or other hypovolaemic conditions because of the risk of inducing hypotension which may be difficult to control. On the other hand a moderate fall in blood pressure due to partial sympathetic block is very common. If treatment is considered desirable, this is best done by increasing the blood volume. Thus an i.v. infusion of 500 (-1000) ml. of a 6 % solution of dextran 70, corresponding to 10 (-20) % of the patient's calculated blood volume, is most suitable.

Sepsis and infection near the pathway of the needle from the skin to the epidural space.

Neurological disease is a relative contraindication. Each case must be judged on its merits.

Fig. 158

COMPLICATIONS

Accidental puncture of the dura – either by needle or catheter. A high or a total spinal will result if the full dose is injected. Therefore a test dose should always be given and the possible effect of this checked.

General toxic symptoms with convulsions, due to too rapid absorption, or injection into the epidural plexus.

Damage to the catheter in the epidural space. The catheter may be removed if it can be found easily at operation, but apparently bits of catheter which have been left in the epidural space do not cause any symptoms even after a long period of observation.

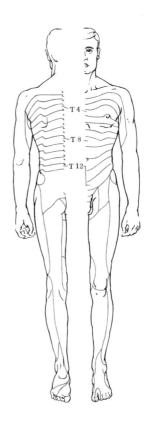

Caudal Anaesthesia

Bertil Löfström

Bertil Löfström

ANATOMY

For caudal anaesthesia a needle is inserted into the epidural space via the *sacral hiatus*. The sacral canal itself is limited dorsally by periosteum covering the four fused sacral spinous processes, with the sacral foramina situated laterally. As a rule the spinous process of the 5th sacral vertebra is not fused, leaving between the two *sacral cornua* an arched opening, the *sacral hiatus,* which is covered by a firm elastic membrane. This ligament partially covers the dorsal surface of the sacrum, lying under the skin and subcutaneous tissue. On the ventral side, the caudal canal is limited by the periosteum and the fused bodies of the sacral vertebrae. The *pelvic sacral foramina* open ventrally towards the ischiorectal fossa, the *dorsal sacral foramina* opening in a backward direction. The epidural space extends right up to the foramen magnum, to which the dura is attached. The coccyx is connected caudally to the sacrum by ligaments (fig. 159).

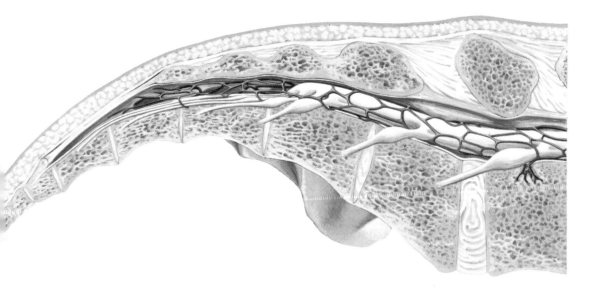

Fig. 159

The epidural space at this level contains nerves from the *cauda equina,* which leave the sacral canal via the pelvic and dorsal sacral foramina. In adults the dural sac extends downwards as far as the second sacral vertebra, i.e. about 1 cm. caudal to a line drawn between the two posterior superior iliac spines.

TECHNIQUE

The patient is placed in the prone position, with the operating table "broken" or with a pillow under the symphysis pubis. The legs are slightly separated with the heels rotated outwards, so as to smooth out the upper part of the anal cleft. In obstetric cases, caudal anaesthesia is performed with the patient in the lateral decubitus (Sim's position) or in the knee-elbow position. A dry gauze swab is placed in the anal cleft, to protect the anal area and genitalia from the spirit used to sterilize the skin.

The posterior superior iliac spines are marked and an equilateral triangle is drawn with its apex pointing caudally (fig. 160). Normally the apex is situated over or immediately adjacent to the sacral hiatus, the cornua of which are palpated and marked. The palpation of these landmarks is best performed if the thumb and middle finger respectively are placed on the spines. Then the index finger is moved caudally in the midline until an equilateral triangle is formed. At this point the two cornua may be located by slightly moving the index finger sideways (fig. 161). The tips of the middle and the index fingers are then placed on the two cornua (fig. 163).

A short, fine-gauge needle (0.50-0.60 mm. in diameter) is inserted in a slightly cranial direction between the tips of the fingers (fig. 163). It is usually easy to feel when the needle pierces the membrane. When the needle has reached the ventral wall of the sacral canal, it is slowly withdrawn whilst 4 ml. of 1 % lignocaine with adrenaline is injected. A further 1 ml. is injected subcutaneously. This produces a block of the

Fig. 160

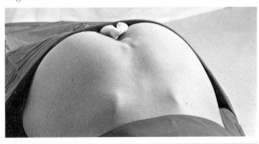

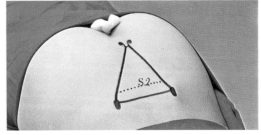

Fig. 161

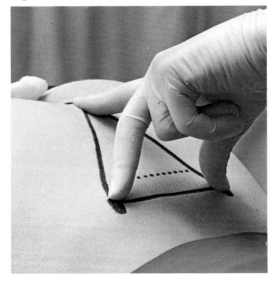

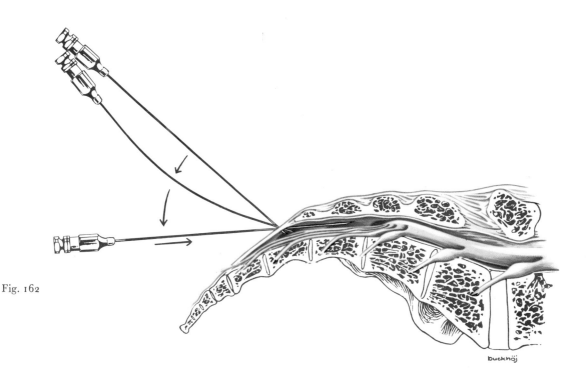

Fig. 162

Fig. 163

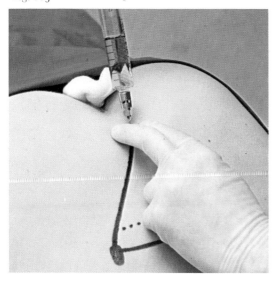

lower sacral nerves resulting in analgesia of the area of the hiatus. By using a fine needle, the sacral canal can usually be entered without discomfort to the patient and without the subcutaneous injection of an appreciable volume of local anaesthetic solution, which would make subsequent palapation more difficult.

A caudal needle or alternatively a rather wide-bored spinal needle (0.90-1.10 mm., i.e. S.W.G. 19-20 or 1.25 mm., i.e. S.W.G. 18, when a catheter technique is employed) is then inserted into the canal along the same tracks as the fine-gauge needle. The orifice of the needle should point in a cranioventral direction. When contact is made with bone

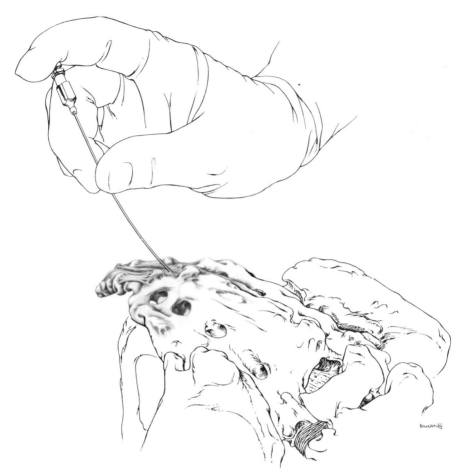

Fig. 164

Fig. 165

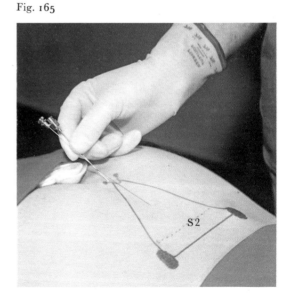

S2

in the sacral canal, the needle is withdrawn slightly and directed more cranially for further insertion into the canal. By bending the needle these two steps may be combined, thus facilitating the insertion of the needle into the sacral extradural space (fig. 162, 164).

The position of the needle in relation to the dura is checked by removing the stilette and holding it immediately above the inserted needle; its point must not reach S 2 (fig. 165). The needle is rotated through $90°$ a couple of times and in the absence of a backflow of cerebrospinal fluid or blood the syringe is attached and aspiration attempted after the needle is further turned through $90°$.

Should a backflow of *cerebro-spinal fluid* be obtained, a local anaesthetic solution for caudal anaesthesia *must not* be injected.

Should *blood* be obtained, the position of the needle is altered until it is certain that it does not lie within a blood vessel.

Should neither blood nor cerebro-spinal fluid be aspirated, local anaesthetic solution is injected slowly whilst the sacral area is palpated. *An injection dorsal to the sacrum* can usually be noted in this way (fig. 166).

Injection should be easy and meet with no resistance. Resistance to injection may indicate *subperiosteal placing of the needle* (fig. 167). In such a case the patient usually experiences considerable pain over the caudal part of the sacrum during the injection. However it should be remembered that slight resistance to injection is quite normal in older patients while the last ml. of a larger volume of local anaesthetic is being injected.

The point of the needle should lie approximately in the midline. If it is placed too far laterally, the risk of puncturing a blood vessel or of obtaining predominantly unilateral analgesia is markedly increased. If the local anaesthetic is injected following previous venipuncture there is a greater risk of toxic reactions, as the solution may be forced into the perforated vessel. Moreover, less satisfactory anaesthesia, often with patchy distribution, is more likely to occur.

TRANS-SACRAL SUPPLEMENTATION

For supplementing a block and in cases where the sacral canal cannot be identified,

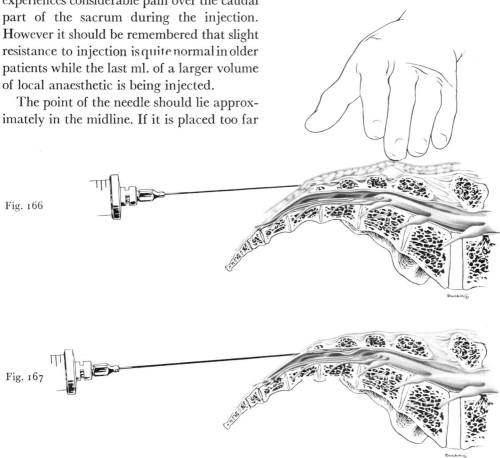

Fig. 166

Fig. 167

137

a needle may be inserted easily through the second sacral foramen. This is situated approximately one finger's breadth medial and caudal to the posterior superior iliac spine. Subcutaneous and periosteal infiltration should be performed. A relatively fine needle, 7-8 cm. long, with a marker, is inserted towards S 2 at right angles to the sacrum. When contact is made with the dorsal surface of the sacrum, the marker is placed 1.5 cm. from the surface of the skin. The needle is moved along the dorsal surface of the sacrum until S 2 is found and then inserted up to the marker.

DOSAGE

The volume of solution injected largely determines the spread of anaesthesia obtained, while its concentration determines the depth of anaesthesia, i.e. the extent to which the coarser myelinated fibres are affected. If 1 % lignocaine with adrenaline is used, a dose of 20 ml. in younger patients or 15 ml. in the more elderly gives a saddle block, extending to the symphysis at the most; 25 ml. will produce a block to the level of T12-T10, in younger patients 30 ml. may be required to provide a block up to the level of T10 etc. The use of a 2 % solution results in somewhat higher levels of anaesthesia but above all, much better muscle relaxation. In addition 1.5-2.0 % solutions provide more rapid onset of anaesthesia. The duration of effect is 2-3 hours. If short anaesthesia is desired i.e. less than 1 hour, lignocaine without added vasoconstrictor should be used.

INDICATIONS

Perineal surgery, painful urological and gynaecological examinations. N.B. For the transurethral removal of ureteric calculi analgesia should extend beyond T 10.

For haemorrhoidectomy, lignocaine with adrenalin 1.5-2 % should be used and analgesia up to a level of T10-T12 is required if considerable rectal traction is to be exerted. It is this which would cause peritoneal pain otherwise.

This form of anaesthesia is also very suitable for use in obstetrics, either as a simple or as a continuous (i.e. intermittent) block. The principles for the catheter technique are the same as with lumbar epidural anaesthesia (cf. p. 125).

Block of the Sympathetic Nervous System - General Considerations

Bertil Löfström

ANATOMICAL SURVEY

The *sympathetic trunk* extends on either side of the vertebral column from the second cervical vertebra down as far as the tip of the coccyx. It consists of a chain of ganglia, which are connected to each other by means of nerve fibres *(the interganglionic rami)*. In the embryonic state, the sympathetic trunk has the same number of ganglia as there are spinal segments (31-32), but in the course of development, the number of ganglia is reduced to between 22 and 24, i.e. 2-3 cervical, 11-12 thoracic, 4 or sometimes 5 lumbar, 4 sacral and 1 coccygeal ganglion.

The sympathetic chain receives both afferent visceral and efferent preganglionic fibres from the thoratic and upper lumbar spinal nerves by way of the *white rami communicantes*. Many of the efferent preganglionic fibres synapse in one or other of the ganglia of the sympathetic chain with the postganglionic neurones. Some of the postganglionic fibres go as *grey rami communicantes* to the spinal nerves, which they then follow to supply the smooth muscle of the blood vessels (vasomotor fibres), the erector muscles of the hair follicles (pilomotor fibres) and the sweat glands (secretor fibres). On the other hand, the preganglionic fibres which supply the viscera pass through the sympathetic chain without synapsing. The synapse with the postganglionic neurones takes place instead in ganglia which lie more peripherally, scattered in a network of autonomic nerves – for example, in *the coeliac plexus and hypogastric plexus.*

GENERAL REMARKS

The peripheral sympathetic fibres run in connective tissue spaces where they lie more or less collected together, although their exact pathway will vary considerably among different individuals. Thus complete block of the sympathetic trunk usually requires that the surrounding connective tissue space be filled with local anaesthetic solution. But on the other hand, a relatively weak solution is required to block the scantily myelinated fibres e.g. 0.5 % lignocaine with adrenaline 1:200,000* for example. Thus sympathetic blocks do not carry great risk of toxic reactions, in spite of the relatively large volume of solution employed.

The sympathetic chain may be blocked both in the region of the neck, or in the lumbar region. Among the visceral plexus *the coeliac* and *the inferior hypogastric plexus* are those where a block may be considered. A direct block of the thoracic sympathetic should not be attempted, because of the great

---

* The use of local anaesthetic solutions containing a vasoconstrictor is considered contraindicated in patients suffering from peripheral vascular disease. In such cases prilocaine or mepivacaine 0.5 % without adrenaline is to be preferred, as these agents give a long-lasting effect even in plain solutions (Albert & Löfström, 1965).

risk of puncture of the lung and subsequent pneumothorax. The fibres from the thoracic sympathetic chain which run cranially may be blocked at *the stellate ganglion*. The nerve supply of the abdominal viscera via the splanchnic nerves may be anaesthetized by means of a coeliac or lumbar sympathetic block.

ASSESSMENT OF SYMPATHETIC BLOCK

It is often difficult to judge whether or not a complete sympathetic block has been obtained, especially when vascular disease is present. A significant increase in warmth, whether subjective or objective, cannot always be registered. Increased filling of the veins is a sign of sympathetic block which is worth looking for, since the venous system is less often the site of pathological changes than the arterial. A positive Horner's syndrome (fig. 173) following a stellate ganglion block is not an indication of a complete sympathetic block of the upper limb and the head. It merely demonstrates that the sympathetic chain in the neck has been blocked.

Objective signs of a complete sympathetic block are an appreciably increased skin temperature compared with the side not block-

ed; an increase in arterial pulsations demonstrated by oscillometry or plethysmography; abolished secretion of sweat in the hand or foot demonstrated by the starch/iodine test, ninhydrin test (Dhunér et al. 1960) as well as the sympathogalvanic reflex (Lewis 1955). This last method is of special value, since the effect of the block can be directly assessed in conjunction with the performance of the block. This test is based upon the fact that pain or emotionally loaded questions result in changes in the electrical resistance of the skin of the hand or foot. These changes are mediated by cholinergic sympathetic fibres and thus are abolished after blocking the sympathetic chain.

The simplest method of eliciting the sympathogalvanic reflex is as follows. Surface electrodes, as used in the recording of ECG, are placed on the palmar and dorsal surfaces of the hands (or on the sole and dorsum of the foot) and connected to the ECG apparatus. The earth lead is attached to an electrode somewhere on the surface of the body (fig. 168).

When the patient has remained undisturbed at rest for a couple of minutes, the ECG apparatus is started. The paper is allowed to run at a fairly slow rate, 5 or 10 mm./sec. for example. When a steady baseline has been established, the patient's skin is pinched. This will change the resistance of the skin between the two electrodes and a deviation of the trace is obtained. With complete sympathetic block, no deflection occurs on the side blocked. In order to be able to evaluate the sympathogalvanic reflex with certainty, a corresponding test should be performed simultaneusly on the side not blocked (Löfström & Thulin 1965). A marked deflection should occur when the skin is pinched so that the effect of the block may be assessed. Note that the patient must not be atropinized prior to this test.

Fig. 168

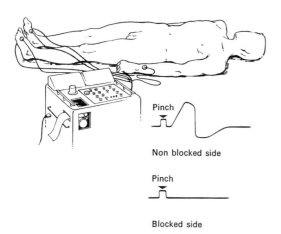

Pinch

Non blocked side

Pinch

Blocked side

Stellate Ganglion Block

Bertil Löfström

ANATOMY

The cervical part of the sympathetic chain is embedded in the *pretracheal lamina* of the cervical fascia and is separted from the transverse processes of the cervical vertebrae by the slender paravertebral musculature. The *vertebral artery* runs upwards in the *transverse foramina* of the transverse processes. The *cervical spinal nerves* are situated in their *spinal nerve sulci,* at first surrounded by the dura and arachnoid. The anterior relations of the cervical sympathetic chain are the *common carotid artery* and, higher up, the *internal carotid artery.* The cervical part of the sympathetic trunk contains only three ganglia, a superior, a middle and a lower. The latter is usually fused with the first thoracic ganglion to form the large *cervicothoracic or stellate ganglion* (fig. 171).

Fig. 169

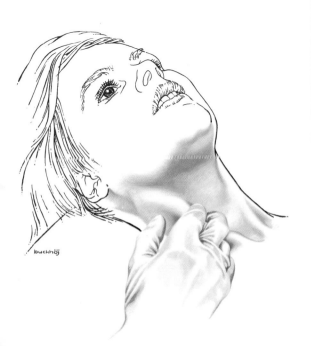

buckhöj

TECHNIQUE

The patient is placed supine, with the head slightly raised and extended backwards on a pillow. With the finger inserted between the sternocleidomastoid muscle and the trachea (fig. 169), the most easily palpated transverse process is sought (usually at a level of the thyroid cartilage – i.e. the 6th). Palpation is facilitated if the patient opens his mouth somewhat. A weal is raised with a fine needle over the transverse process. Using two fingers, the anaesthetist presses down the skin between the sternocleido-mastoid muscle and the common carotid artery on one side and the thyroid, trachea and oesophagus on the other side. One finger should palpate the transverse process and at the same time allowing the insertion of a finegauge needle, 5-8 cm. long, towards this transverse process until it makes contact with it (fig. 170).

Note that the needle during its insertion must not penetrate any tissue which offers appreciable resistance. It is, in fact, easy to insert the needle by mistake through membrane, muscle attachments or muscles ex-

Fig. 170

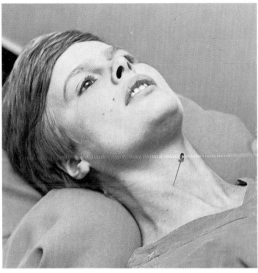

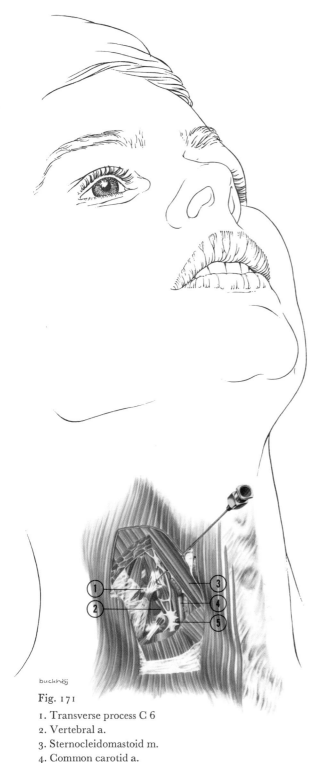

Fig. 171

1. Transverse process C 6
2. Vertebral a.
3. Sternocleidomastoid m.
4. Common carotid a.
5. Stellate ganglion

tending between the transverse processes. If this were to happen the needle could easily puncture the vertebral artery or contact bone *inside* the spinal nerve sulci, possibly resulting in a puncture of the dural cuff, which emerges through the intervertebral foramen.

When the needle rests upon the transverse process, the palpating fingers are drawn up. Then the point of the needle is withdrawn a few millimetres and fixed. After careful aspiration, 15-20 ml. of lignocaine, mepivacaine or prilocaine 0.5 % with or without adrenaline are injected (fig. 171). This relatively large volume is required in order to fill the fascial compartment anterior to the vertebral column containing the network of sympathetic fibres (fig. 172 a, b).

A positive Horner's syndrome (fig. 173), (ptosis, myosis, enopthalmosis, anhydrosis) occuring with block of the stellate ganglion is not an indication of complete block of the sympathetic innervation of the upper extremity and head. It merely demonstrates that the sympathetic chain in the neck has been blocked (cf. p. 140).

If a series of sympathetic blocks are planned, it is usually an advantage to give the first injection at the level of C6. Should a haematoma appear, it is then usually possible to produce a satisfactory block by placing the needle against the transverse process of C7.

INDICATIONS

The indications for stellate ganglion block are mainly regional circulatory insufficiency and sympathetic (visceral) pain. Clinical conditions in which stellate ganglion block is of value are Reynaud's disease (temporarily); arterial embolism, when oedema, swelling and pain are present in conjunction with the so-called post-traumatic syndrome; in cases of vascular injury or vascular surgery on the upper limb and in patients suffering from severe angina pectoris.

In order to obtain therapeutic effect a series of blocks is usually required, e.g. one block each day over a period of 4-5 days, followed by a block every other day, repeated four or five times. Simultaneous bilateral stellate ganglion block should be avoided, as a rule, because of the risk of complications.

Stellate ganglion block should be combined with other conventional forms of treatment such as physiotherapy, protection from cold, etc.

COMPLICATIONS

Haematoma occurs fairly readily and hampers subsequent blocks, but requires no special treatment. *Recurrent nerve paralysis* or *partial involvement of the brachial plexus* may occur, but require no treatment.

Intravascular injection of an appreciable amount of local anaesthetic solution, especially into the vertebral artery, should be prevented by repeated aspiration, the needle being rotated between each attempt. Moreover, the injection should always be administered slowly, the patient being watched carefully for any sign of toxic reaction to the local anaesthetic agent such as dizziness or unconsciousness.

Puncture of the dura cannot, as a rule, be diagnosed by the spontaneous backflow of cerebro-spinal fluid, or by aspiration, because the hydrostatic pressure in the dural cuffs protruding through the intervertebral foramina is low. Furthermore, the dura itself is very thin here and may easily occlude the aperture of the needle. The subarachnoid injection of 15-20 ml. 0.5 % solution of lignocaine, prilocaine or mepivacaine would result in widespread spinal anaesthesia, commencing in the cervical region, where it would be most intense.

Osteitis in the transverse process is a rare complication. This could possibly be due to the oesophagus having been perforated by the needle as it approached the transverse process.

Mediastinitis, with formation of gravitation intrathoracic abscess has been described in the literature.

Pleural puncture with pneumothorax need not be feared if the technique described above is carefully carried out.

Fig. 172 a   Fig. 172 b

Fig. 173

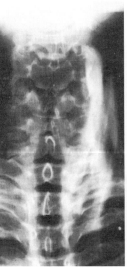

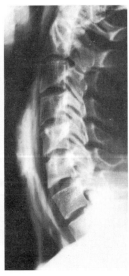
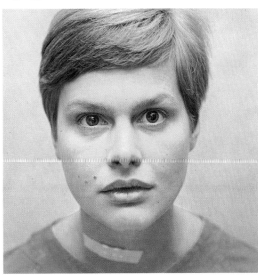

Lumbar Sympathetic Block

Bertil Löfström

ANATOMY

The *sympathetic chain* with its ganglia is located on the ventrolateral aspect of the vertebral bodies in a fascial compartment limited by the vertebral column, the psoas sheath and the retroperitoneal fascia. This space is closed cranially at the level of the body of the first lumbar vertebra. A sympathetic block of this chain using conventional local anaesthetic agents merely requires the tip of the needle to be placed from the dor-

sum into this space. However, when a so-called chemical sympathectomy is to be performed, using a small volume of phenol or alcohol, the point of the needle must lie immediately adjacent to the sympathetic chain (fig. 174).

The landmarks which are used for the performance of this block are as follows: L1 which is situated at the level of the junction of the 12th rib and the erector spinae muscles and L4-L5 at the level of a line drawn between the two posterior iliac crests (fig. 175).

SINGLE SHOT TECHNIQUE

Preferably the patient should lie in the lateral position with the waist supported either by a pillow or by "breaking" the table so that the vertebral column is curved in a lateral plane and the spaces between the transverse processes are widened out on the upper side. Weals are raised opposite the

Fig. 174

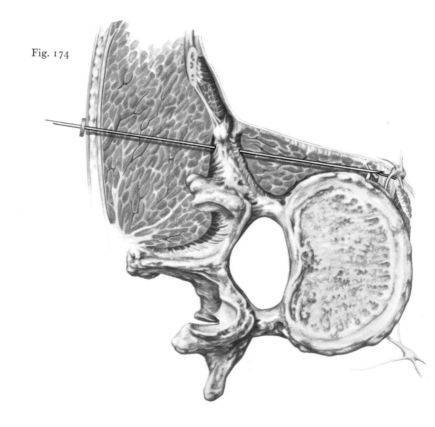

spinous processes of L2 and L4, 7-10 cm. lateral to the mid-line. A 19 S.W.G. needle 12-18 cm. long,* with a marker on it, is introduced through the weal and directed 45° cranially or caudally so that it strikes the transverse process of the vertebra lying above or below it (fig. 176). On making contact with bone the marker is pushed down to the skin and the needle withdrawn. If the patient is of normal size, the marker is moved so that its position from the point equals double the distance between the skin and the transverse process (fig. 177). In thin patients, the length of needle to be introduced should be slightly increased but in stout patients slightly decreased. This distance from the tip of the needle to the marker will correspond roughly to the distance between the skin and the ventero-lateral aspect of the vertebral bodies. The needle is now inserted be-

tween the transverse processes and directed more medially, but at right angles to the skin, in the sagittal plane. This space will be found approximately opposite the corresponding spinous process. If the needle strikes bone when the marker is close to the skin, the point will be in contact with the lateral aspect of the body of the vertebra (fig. 176). The bevel of the needle should face the body of the vertebra to that slight bending of the needle will allow it to slip forwards to lie adjacent to the sympathetic chain. A minor adjustment of the position of the needle may be necessary. The position of the needle may be checked by X-ray (cf. chemical sympathectomy p. 147).

Complete sympathetic block may be obtained either by using a single injection at the level of L2, using 25-30 ml. of 0.5 % mepivacaine or prilocaine. However, it is even better to use two needles, one being inserted at L2 and the other at L4 and to inject 15 ml. of

* Becton, Dickinson and Co., Rutherford, New Jersey.

Fig. 175

Fig. 176

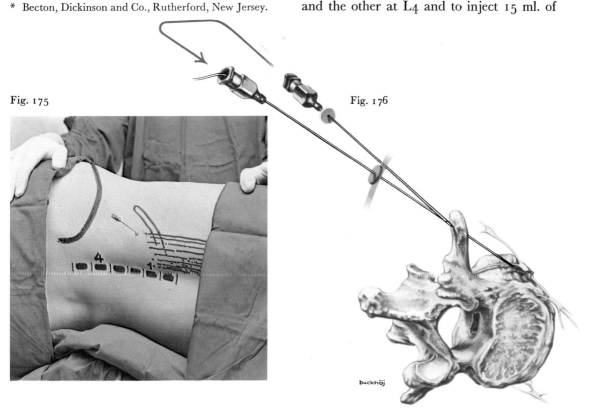

buckhöj

the same solution through each needle (fig. 178). A solution without vasoconstrictor should be used for patients suffering from peripheral vascular disease. For treatment of pain (e.g. nephrolithiasis), solutions containing a vasoconstrictor should be employed.

The following simplified technique may be used when a "one-shot" block is to be performed: After adjustment of the marker as previously described, the needle is reinserted somewhat nearer the mid-line than recommended above. The angle to the mid-line should also be reduced. If the needle is pushed up to the marker, injecting the local anaesthetic solution even if bone contact has not been made usually results in satisfactory lumbar sympathetic block. This technique should not, however, be employed for continuous lumbar sympathetic block or for chemical sympathectomy.

CONTINUOUS TECHNIQUE

When a continuous block using an indwelling catheter is to be performed, somewhat wider needles than for a simple block, i.e. 18 S.W.G. are used. Their lumen should be of such a diameter that the vinyl or teflon catheters can be threaded easily. This should be checked before the needles are inserted. When the needle has been inserted into its correct position as described above, the catheter is threaded through it until a slight resistance is met indicating that the tip of the needle has been reached (fig. 179). The catheter is then pushed in approximately 1 cm. further. While the needle is carefully withdrawn the catheter is fed simultaneously through it for an equivalent distance. This usually results in an additional centimetre or two of the catheter being curled up in the tissues. Fig. 180 shows the

Fig. 177

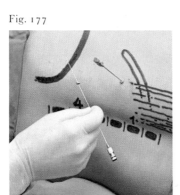

Fig. 178

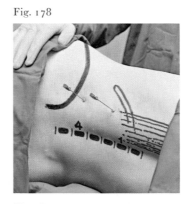

Fig. 179

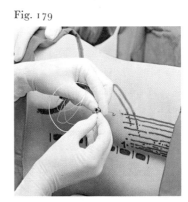

Fig. 180

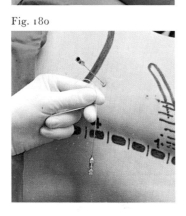

Fig. 181

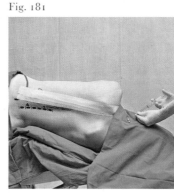

Fig. 182

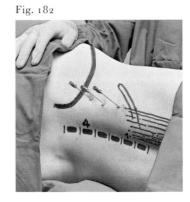

situation following the introduction of the catheter. If the catheter does not slide easily into place it must be withdrawn together with the needle and the whole procedure recommenced.

The sites where the catheters emerge are covered with adhesive tape and the catheters are fixed to the skin overlying the erector spinae muscles (N.B. Not over the spinous processes, where tissue damage from pressure may easily occur). Preferably they should be drawn up over the shoulder and lie in the supraclavicular fossa where short-bevelled needles with stoppers are inserted into the open ends (fig. 181). These needles should then be rolled up in gauze soaked in antiseptic and wrapped up in a sterile swab. Every four hours 10-15 ml. mepivacaine or prilocaine 0.5 % are injected through each catheter. It is considered that solutions containing a vasoconstrictor should not be administered to patients suffering from peripheral vascular disease. In such patients prilocaine and mepivacaine are to be recommended, since these drugs produce relatively long lasting anaesthesia even without the addition of adrenaline (Albért & Löfström 1965). The catheters should not be left in position for longer than 4 or 5 days. Decreasing effect of the block may be due to dislocation of a catheter. This can be demonstrated by means of X-ray, injecting a few ml. of water soluble contrast solution (fig. 183 a, b).

CHEMICAL SYMPATHECTOMY

The points of three needles are placed against the bodies of L2, L3, L4 (fig. 182). Their positions are checked by X-rays. In the lateral view, the needle points should barely reach the anterior borders of the vertebral bodies (fig. 184 a) and in the anteroposterior view they should lie over them. Thus in fig. 184 b the needles have not yet reached their correct position. When they are in place, 3 ml. of 6.5-7 % phenol dissolved in water, or 3 ml. of absolute alcohol, are injected through each needle.

INDICATIONS

Peripheral Vascular Disease: Sympathetic blockade is considered to be of value in cases of incipient gangrene, especially if the

Fig. 183 a Fig. 183 b

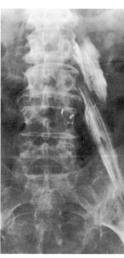 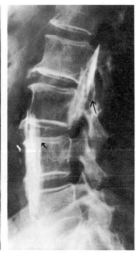

Fig. 184 a Fig. 184 b

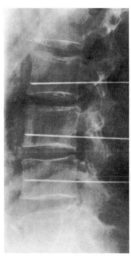 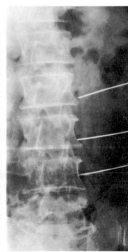

147

pathological changes in the blood-vessels are not too widespread. In widespread vascular disease, sympathetic block may cause an impaired blood-flow through the partially occluded vessels if the circulation in the more proximal vascular bed and the skin is markedly increased. Consequently unilateral sympathetic block may well be better than bilateral block obtained by epidural anaesthesia.

Phenol blockade may be of value also in cases of intermittent claudication with limited occlusion situated proximally. However, such patients should be assessed carefully prior to chemical sympathectomy, especially regarding the possibility of reconstructive vascular surgery (Löfström & Zetterquist, 1967).

Treatment of Painful Conditions: Patients suffering from nephrolithiasis with colic respond particularly well to this treatment. However, the pathways of pain of the renal pelvis are not always blocked adequately by this method. A block at the level of L1 often gives better results than those at the levels of L2 and L4. Should the renal pelvis be accidentally punctured, it should be emptied of urine before the needle is withdrawn and the needle reinserted in a different position.

COMPLICATIONS

A *fall in blood-pressure* occurs frequently in elderly patients with severe vascular disease. Therefore the author always sets up a slow intravenous drip of 500 ml. of dextran 40 before the block is performed. Should the blood-pressure begin to fall the drip rate is speeded up. Usually this measure is sufficient to stabilise the blood-pressure at an acceptable level. N.B. Never tilt the patient head-down except when vitally necessary. This position, in combination with a low blood-pressure, predisposes to thrombosis in diseased vessels of the lower limbs. If there is a marked fall in pressure, the volume of local anaesthetic used for repeated doses should be reduced.

Intravascular injection is avoided by aspiration.

Paraesthesiae occuring while the needle is being inserted are relatively common. The easiest way to avoid this complication is to insert the needle a fair distance from the mid-line.

Subarachnoid injection can occur, should the needle be directed too far medially and the anaesthetist not appreciate the significance of bone contact being made too superficially. In such a case the needle slipping in through the intervertebral foramen is confused by the anaesthetist with the sensation of its slipping off the verterolateral aspect of the vertebral body.

Bleeding in the psoas sheath manifests itself as pain radiating to the groin and the upper medial part of the thigh, together with pain on rotation in the hip joint. Such bleeding may be lethal if a sympathetic block is attempted in a heparinized patient. Heparin administration must, therefore, be considered an absolute contraindication to sympathetic block. In the author's experience, significant bleeding does not occur if the prothrombin-proconventin index is reduced to 12-15 % by the administration of anticoagulants of the dicoumaral group.

Neuritis, involving especially the genitofemoral nerve which runs in the psoas sheath, may easily occur following chemical sympathectomy.

Local anaesthesia for arthroscopy

EJNAR ERIKSSON

Although epidural or spinal anaesthesia seem to offer advantages for the performance of arthroscopy it is the author's experience that a large percentage of all arthroscopies can be performed with local anaesthesia. This allows the examined patient to return home immediately after the investigation.

TECHNIQUE

5–10 cc of 0.5 % lignocaine or prilocaine with vasoconstrictor is infiltrated at the anterior site of insertion of the arthroscope. The skin and the underlying tissues down to the joint capsule are anesthestized (fig. 185).

A second skin weal is raised just above and lateral to the upper lateral corner of the patella. The skin and underlying tissues are infiltrated down to the joint capsule. Another 5–10 cc of 0.5 % lignocaine or prilocaine with vasoconstrictor are used for this. A 50 cc syringe with a large bore needle is then used to fill the knee joint with 50 cc of 0.5 % lignocaine or prilocaine with vasoconstrictor through this upper anaesthetic weal (fig. 186). The patient is then asked to move his knee joint for a couple of minutes. After about 5 minutes the arthroscope can be inserted through the previously anaesthetized (and marked) area. When the arthroscope is inside the joint this is further dilated by the injection of a mixture of 5 cc of 0.5 % lignocaine or prilocaine with vasoconstrictor and 45 cc of physiological saline through the arthroscope (fig. 187). The arthroscopy is thereafter carried out in this diluted anaesthetized drug through the two anaesthetized areas. If further fluid needs to be injected a mixture of 5 cc 0.5 % lignocaine or prilocaine with vasoconstrictor and 45 cc of physiological saline is used.

Fig. 185. A skin wheal is raised at the site of entry of the arthroscope. The underlying tissues down to the joint capsule are injected with 6–10 ml of 0.5 % prilocaine or lignocaine. One should avoid injecting too much into the fat pad since this will diminish visibility inside the knee joint. Fig. 186. After the skin proximal and lateral to the patella has been anaesthetized a large bore needle is inserted into the supra patellar pouch and 50 ml of 0.5 % prilocaine or lignocaine is injected. The knee is then moved 7–8 times so that the anaesthetic is evenly distributed within the knee joint. One should allow 4–5 minutes for the anaesthetic to take.

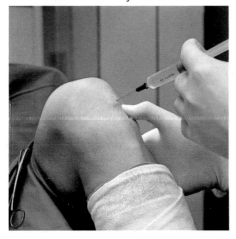 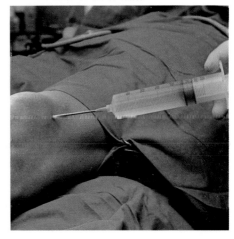

The presence of local anaesthetic in the joint does not interfere with the picture quality (fig 188).

It has been claimed that the use of vasoconstrictors should cause a "white-out" of the knee joint capsule. This has not been the finding of the author. The vasoconstrictor has eliminated bleeding from the puncture sites and thereby reduced the need for continuous flushing of the joint. It has caused very little bleaching of the capsule. It has always been possible to judge the degree of synovitis.

The patients have often been able to walk off the examining table themselves. They have been allowed to return home after a couple of hours observation.

DOSAGE

70–100 cc of 0.5 % lignocaine or prilocaine with 1:200.000 vasoconstrictor often needs to be used. Determination of blood concentrations of prilocaine after this procedure (Eriksson & Al – to be published) has shown the method to be very safe.

INDICATIONS

Out patient arthroscopy for diagnostic or therapeutic purposes. It is also possible to remove loose bodies or perform a partial meniscectomy with the use of this anaesthetic technique.

Any arthroscope can be used. The author has routinely been using a 5 mm Storz arthroscope. It is sometimes said that arthroscopy under local anaesthesia can only be performed with the help of small diameter, socalled "needle-scope". With the technique described here it is possible to use even 6–7 mm operating arthroscopes.

CONTRAINDICATIONS

Very anxious patients and children below 15 years. The choice of anaesthesia should be discussed with the patient prior to the examination. It should be explained to him that he might feel when the arthroscope is moved inside the joint but that he will not feel any pain.

Local anaesthesia should be avoided in patients that claim that they have reacted unfavourably to local anaesthesia previously.

Fig. 187. When the arthroscope has been inserted the knee is further distended with a mixture of 5–10 ml of 0.5 % prilocaine or lignocaine and 40–45 ml of physiological saline. The examination is thus carried out in a dilute local anaesthetic solution. Fig. 188. Arthroscopic picture of an acute rupture of the anterior cruciate ligament photographed with the joint distended with prilocaine. Local anaesthesia can also be used in acute arthroscopies after the haemarthrosis has been washed out with physiological saline.

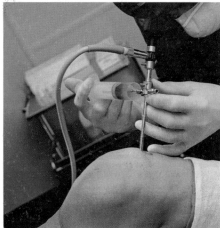
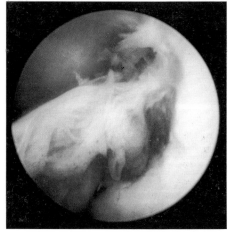

References

This list contains the literature specially referred to in the various chapters. However, it does not claim to be complete, nor even a cross section of the literature in the field of local anaesthesia.

ADAMS, J. P., E. J. DEALY & P. I. KENMORE: Intravenous Regional Anesthesia in Hand Surgery. J. Bone Jt. Surg. *46-A*, 811, 1964.

ADRIANI, J., R. ZEPERNICK & E. HYDE: Influence of the Status of the Patient on Systemic Effects of Local Anesthetic Agents. Anesth. Analg. Curr. Res. *45*, 87, 1966.

ALBÉRT, J. & B. LÖFSTRÖM: Bilateral Ulnar Nerve Blocks for the Evaluation of Local Anaesthetic Agents. Acta anaesth. scand. *5*, 99, 1961.

ALBÉRT, J. & B. LÖFSTRÖM: Bilateral Ulnar Nerve Blocks for the Evaluation of Local Anaesthetic Agents. II. Acta anaesth. scand. *9*, 1, 1965 (a).

ALBÉRT, J. & B. LÖFSTRÖM: Bilateral Ulnar Nerve Blocks for the Evaluation of Local Anaesthetic Agents. III. Acta anaesth. scand. *9*, 203, 1965 (b).

ANTONI, N.: Comments on Neurological Diagnosis by Puncture. Acta psychiat. scand., suppl. 59, 1948.

ARNER, O.: Complications Following Spinal Anaesthesia, Their Significance and a Technic to Reduce Their Incidence. Acta chir. scand., suppl. 167, 1952.

BELL, H. M., E. M. SLATER & W. H. HARRIS: Regional Anesthesia with Intravenous Lidocaine. J. Amer. med. Ass. *186*, 544, 1963.

BERGMAN, P. & T. MALMSTRÖM: Lokalanestesi med Xylocain-spray som ersättning för slutnarkos vid förlossning och som anestesimetod vid perineotomier. Svenska Läk.-Tidn. *58*, 2359, 1961.

BERGMAN, P. & T. MALMSTRÖM: Örtliche Betäubung mit Xylocain als geburtshilfliche Anästhesiemethode. Geburtsh. u. Frauenheilk. *23*, 136, 1963.

BERNHARD, C. G. & E. BOHM: Local Anaesthetics as Anticonvulsants. Almqvist & Wiksell, Stockholm, 1965.

BIER, A.: Ueber einen neuen Weg Localanästhesie an den Gliedmaassen zu erzeugen. Arch. klin. Chir. *86*, 1007, 1908.

BONICA, J. J., P. H. BACKUP, C. E. ANDERSON, D. HADFIELD, W. F. CREPPS & B. F. MONK: Peridural Block – Analysis of 3,637 Cases and a Review. Anesthesiology *18*, 723, 1957.

BROMAGE, P. R.: Spinal Epidural Analgesia. E. & S. Livingstone Ltd., Edinburgh and London, 1954.

BROMAGE, P. R.: Spread af Analgesic Solutions in the Epidural Space and Their Site of Action – A Statistical Study. Brit. J. Anaesth. *34*, 161, 1962.

BROMAGE, P. R.: Physiology and Pharmacology of Epidural Analgesia. Anesthesiology *28*, 592, 1967.

BROWN, E. M. & F. WEISSMAN: A Case Report – Prolonged Intravenous Regional Anesthesia. Anesth. Analg. Curr. Res. *45*, 319, 1966.

DHUNÉR, K. G., S. EDSHAGE & A. WILHELM: Ninhydrin Test – An Objective Method for Testing Local Anaesthetic Drugs. Acta anaesth. scand. *4*, 189, 1960.

EDLING, N. P. G.: Urethrocystography in the Male with Special Regard to Micturition. Acta radiol., suppl. 58, 1945.

ERIKSSON, E.: Axillary Brachial plexus anaesthesia in children with citanest. Acta anaesth. scand. Suppl. XVI, 291–296.

ERIKSSON, E., A. PERSSON & B. ÖRTENGREN: Intravenous Regional Anaesthesia – An Attempt to Determine the Safety of the Method and a Comparison between Prilocaine and Lidocaine. Acta chir. scand., suppl. 358, 47, 1966.

FRANKSSON, C. & T. GORDH: Headache after Spinal Anesthesia and a Technique for Lessening Its Frequency. Acta chir. scand. *94*, 443, 1946.

FRIEDEN, J.: Antiarrhythmic Drugs. Part VII. Lidocaine as an Antiarrhythmic Agent. Amer. Heart J. *70*, 713, 1965.

GEDDES, J. S., A. A. J. ADGEY & J. F. PANTRIDGE: Prognosis after Recovery from Ventricular Fibrillation Complicating Ischaemic Heart-Disease. Lancet II, 273, 1967.

GEJROT, T.: Intravenous Xylocaine in the Treatment of Attacks of Menière's Disease. Acta oto-laryng. (Stockh.), suppl. 188, 190, 1963 (a).

GEJROT, T.: The Influence of Xylocaine on Induced and Spontaneous Nystagmus. Pract. oto-rhino-laryng. *25*, 361, 1963 (b).

GIANELLY, R., J. O. VON DER GROEBEN, A. P. SPIVACK & D. C. HARRISON: Effect of Lidocaine on Ventricular Arrhythmias in Patients with Coronary Heart Disease. New Engl. J. Med. *277*, 1215, 1967.

GORDH, T.: Intravenous Barbiturate Anaesthesia in the Treatment of Convulsions due to Local Anaesthesia. Proc. 2nd Congress Scand. Soc. Anaesth. 1952.

GORDH, T.: Heart-Volume Studies I-III. I. Pneumopericardium as Plethysmograph for Cardiometry in the Rabbit. Acta anaesth. scand. *8*, 1, 1964 (a).

GORDH, T.: Heart-Volume Studies I-III. II. Effect of Various Anaesthetics and Drugs on the Heart Volume in the Rabbit. Acta anaesth. scand. *8*, 15, 1964 (b).

GORDH, T. & Å. LILJESTRAND: Om giftigheten hos lokalanestetika. Svenska Läk.-Tidn. *43*, 1885, 1946.

GROSSMAN, J. I., L. A. LUBOW, J. FRIEDEN & I. L. RUBIN: Lidocaine in Cardiac Arrhythmias. Arch. intern. Med. *121*, 396, 1968.

HARRISON, D. C., J. H. SPROUSE & A. G. MORROW: The Antiarrhythmic Properties of Lidocaine and Procaine Amide. Circulation 28, 486, 1963.

HOLMBERG, S.: Personal communication.

HOLMES, C. McK.: Intravenous Regional Analgesia. A Useful Method of Producing Analgesia of the Limbs. Lancet I, 245, 1963.

JEWITT, D. E., R. BALCON, E. B. RAFTERY & S. ORAM: Incidence and Management of Supraventricular Arrhythmias after Acute Myocardial Infarction. Lancet II, 734, 1967.

KLINGENSTRÖM, P.: The Effect of Ergotamine on Blood Pressure, Epecially in Spinal Anaesthesia. Acta anaesth. scand., suppl. 4, 1960.

LEWIS, L. L.: Evaluation of Sympathetic Activity Following Chemical or Surgical Sympathectomy. Anesth. Analg. Curr. Res. 34, 334, 1955.

LIKOFF, W.: Editorial. Cardiac Arrhythmias Complicating Surgery. Amer. J. Cardiol. 3, 427, 1959.

LILJEDAHL, S.-O.: Prolongation of Tetracaine (Pontocaine) Spinal Anaesthesia by Supplementary Noradrenaline, with Special Reference to Its Mode of Action. Acta. chir. scand., suppl. 202, 1955.

LÖFSTRÖM, B.: To be published.

LÖFSTRÖM, B. & L. THULIN: Procedures for Objective Evaluation of Nerve Blocks. Acta anaesth. scand. 9, 213, 1965.

LÖFSTRÖM, B. & S. ZETTERQUIST: The Effect of Lumbar Sympathetic Block upon the Nutritive Blood-Flow Capacity in Intermittent Claudication. A Metabolic Study. Acta med. scand. 182, 23, 1967.

LOWN, B., A. M. FAKHRO, W. B. HOOD & G. W. THORN: The Coronary Care Unit. New Perspectives and Directions. J. Amer. med. Ass. 199, 188, 1967.

MERRIFIELD, A. J. & S. J. CARTER: Intravenous Regional Analgesia: Lignocaine Blood Levels. Anaesthesia 20, 287, 1965.

MOBERG, E. & F. W. RATHKE: Dringliche Handchirurgie. Georg Thieme Verlag, Stuttgart, 1964.

MOORE, D. C. & L. D. BRIDENBAUGH: Intercostal Nerve Block in 4,333 Patients: Indications, Technique and Complications. Anesth. Analg. Curr. Res. 41, 1, 1962.

OCHOTSKIJ, W. P.: Intraossale Novocainanästhesie bei Operationen an Extremitäten. Beitr. Orthop. Traum. 8, 138, 1961.

OLIVER, M. F., D. G. JULIAN & K. W. DONALD: Problems in Evaluating Coronary Care Units. Their Responsibilities and Their Relation to the Community. Amer. J. Cardiol. 20, 465, 1967.

ORLOV, G. A.: Intraosseous Anaesthesia during Plastic Operations of the Hand and Fingers. Acta Chir. plast. 2, 59, 1960.

ROSSBERG, G.: Die Unterscheidung peripherer und zentraler Vestibularisstörungen durch die experimentellen Gleichgewichtsprüfungen. Arch. Ohr.-, Nas.-, u. Kehlk.-Heilk. 183, 133, 1965.

SKOOG TORD: Plastic Surgery. Stockholm 1974. Boston 1973.

SMITH, R. M.: Anesthesia for Infants and Children. 3rd Ed., The C. V. Mosby Company, S:t Louis, 1968.

STEINHAUS, J. E.: Local Anaesthetic Toxicity: A Pharmacological Re-Evaluation. Anesthesiology 18, 275, 1957.

TELIVUO, L.: A New Long-Acting Local Anaesthetic Solution for Pain Relief after Thoracotomy. Ann. Chir. Gynaec. Fenn. 52, 513, 1963.

Index

Thiopentone, 14, 18, 21, 22, 94

Throat, local anesthesia of, 39, 42

Thyroid, surgery, local anaesthesia for, 43, 78

Thyrotoxicosis,
adrenaline content of local anaesthetic solutions, 43, 44
cervical plexus block, 78
infiltration anaesthesia for thyroid surgery, 43, 78
premedication, 22

Tibial nerve, block of, 112

Toe, block of, 50

Tonometry, surface anaesthesia for, 26

Tonsillectomy, local anaesthesia for, 42

Toxic reactions, see Reactions due to local anaesthetics

Toxicity of local anaesthetics, see Local anaesthetic agents

Tracheoscopy, surface anaesthesia for, 39

Trans-sacral supplementation of caudal anaesthesia, 137

Trigeminal nerve
anatomy, 58
block of branches, 64, 6, 71

Tympanic membrane, anaesthesia of, 33, 35

U

Ulnar nerve, block of, 86, 91

Urethra, anaesthesia of,
caudal anesthesia, 138
epidural anaesthesia, 131
spinal anaesthsia, 118, 123
surface anaesthesia, 55

V

Vacuum extraction, see Paracervical block and Pudendal nerve block

Varicose veins, nerve block for operations on, 105, 107, 111, 122, 131

Vascular insufficiency, peripheral, relief by sympathetic block, 131, 139, 142, 147

Vasoconstrictor,
addition to local anaesthetics, 11, 12, 13, 43, 44, 96, 97, 100, 118, 139, 147

Vaso-vagal reflex, prevention by atropine, 20

W

Wrist, nerve block at, 90